T0269210

CAMBRIDGE LIBRARY COLLECTION

Books of enduring scholarly value

History of Medicine

It is sobering to realise that as recently as the year in which On the Origin of Species was published, learned opinion was that diseases such as typhus and cholera were spread by a 'miasma', and suggestions that doctors should wash their hands before examining patients were greeted with mockery by the profession. The Cambridge Library Collection reissues milestone publications in the history of Western medicine as well as studies of other medical traditions. Its coverage ranges from Galen on anatomical procedures to Florence Nightingale's common-sense advice to nurses, and includes early research into genetics and mental health, colonial reports on tropical diseases, documents on public health and military medicine, and publications on spa culture and medicinal plants.

Reports of a Series of Inoculations for the Variolae Vaccinae or Cowpox

The physician and botanist William Woodville (1752–1805), a proponent of inoculation against smallpox, was in 1791 appointed physician to the London Smallpox and Inoculation Hospital. Five years later, Edward Jenner announced his experiments with vaccination – inoculation with the much milder cowpox, which conveyed immunity to smallpox without the attendant risk of catching the often fatal disease. Woodville eagerly pursued trials using vaccination, and published the results in this 1799 work, which describes two hundred cases where patients (usually children) were vaccinated with matter obtained from either cows or other cowpox sufferers, and supplies a table of the patterns of infection from person to person. Most of these patients were later tested by inoculation with smallpox, and none caught the disease. This demonstration of the safety and efficacy of vaccination led to its much wider adoption, to which Woodville gave practical support in both England and France.

Cambridge University Press has long been a pioneer in the reissuing of out-of-print titles from its own backlist, producing digital reprints of books that are still sought after by scholars and students but could not be reprinted economically using traditional technology. The Cambridge Library Collection extends this activity to a wider range of books which are still of importance to researchers and professionals, either for the source material they contain, or as landmarks in the history of their academic discipline.

Drawing from the world-renowned collections in the Cambridge University Library and other partner libraries, and guided by the advice of experts in each subject area, Cambridge University Press is using state-of-the-art scanning machines in its own Printing House to capture the content of each book selected for inclusion. The files are processed to give a consistently clear, crisp image, and the books finished to the high quality standard for which the Press is recognised around the world. The latest print-on-demand technology ensures that the books will remain available indefinitely, and that orders for single or multiple copies can quickly be supplied.

The Cambridge Library Collection brings back to life books of enduring scholarly value (including out-of-copyright works originally issued by other publishers) across a wide range of disciplines in the humanities and social sciences and in science and technology.

Reports of a Series of Inoculations for the Variolae Vaccinae or Cowpox

*With Remarks and Observations on This Disease,
Considered as a Substitute for the Smallpox*

WILLIAM WOODVILLE

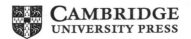

CAMBRIDGE
UNIVERSITY PRESS

CAMBRIDGE
UNIVERSITY PRESS

University Printing House, Cambridge, CB2 8BS, United Kingdom

Cambridge University Press is part of the University of Cambridge.
It furthers the University's mission by disseminating knowledge in the pursuit of
education, learning and research at the highest international levels of excellence.

www.cambridge.org
Information on this title: www.cambridge.org/9781108077699

© in this compilation Cambridge University Press 2017

This edition first published 1799
This digitally printed version 2017

ISBN 978-1-108-07769-9 Paperback

REPORTS

OF A

SERIES OF INOCULATIONS

FOR THE

VARIOLÆ VACCINÆ,

OR

COW-POX;

WITH

REMARKS AND OBSERVATIONS ON THIS
DISEASE, CONSIDERED AS A SUBSTITUTE FOR
THE

SMALL-POX.

By WILLIAM WOODVILLE, M. D.

PHYSICIAN TO THE SMALL-POX AND INOCULATION HOSPITALS.

London:

PRINTED AND SOLD BY

James Phillips and Son,

GEORGE-YARD, LOMBARD-STREET.

1799.

Sir,

The great attention with which you honoured some of the first cases described in the following sheets, has induced me to hope, that an account of the whole, though not affording the satisfactory evidence upon the subject that I expected, may still not be entirely unacceptable to you.

I have the honour to be,
With the utmost regard,
Your obedient Servant,

W. WOODVILLE.

Ely-Place,
May 16th, 1799.

REPORTS, &c.

LAST Summer Dr. JENNER prefented to the public * feveral curious and interefting facts, refpecting a difeafe known to dairy farmers by the name of Cow-pox. The moft important of thefe is, that perfons who have been affected with this diftemper are thereby rendered as fecure from the effects of the variolous infection as if they had actually undergone the Small-pox.

* See an Inquiry into the caufes and effects of the Variolæ vaccinæ, a difeafe difcovered in fome of the Weftern counties of England, particularly Glouceflerfhire, and known by the name of the Cow-pox.

However

However extraordinary this circumſtance may appear, it is ſupported by numerous experiments made under Dr. Jenner's in-ſpection, and alſo by concurrent teſtimonies ſince collated by Dr. Pearſon, † who with much laudable zeal and induſtry inſtituted a farther inquiry into the ſubject.

Dr. Jenner, who from his ſituation, in Glouceſterſhire, had many opportunities of ſeeing the Cow-pox, ſuppoſes it to originate from the matter of the greaſe in horſes, and to take place in the following manner:

" In this dairy-country a great number of cows are kept, and the office of milking is performed indiſcriminately by men and maid ſervants. One of the former having been appointed to apply dreſſings to the heels of a horſe affected with *the greaſe,* and not paying due attention to cleanlinefs, incautioufly bears his part in milking the cows, with fome particles of the infectious matter adhering to his fingers. When this is the cafe, it commonly happens that a difeafe is communicated to the cows, and from the cows to the dairy-maids, which fpreads through the farm, until moft of the cattle and domeftics feel its unpleafant confequences. This difeafe has obtained the name of the Cow-pox. It appears on the nipples of the cows, in the form of irregular puftules. At their firft appearance they are commonly of a palifh blue, or rather of a colour fomewhat approaching to livid, and are furrounded by an eryfipelatous inflammation. Thefe puftules, unlefs a timely remedy be applied, frequently degenerate into phagedenic ulcers. The animals become indifpofed, and the fecretion of milk is much leffened. Inflamed fpots now begin to appear on different

A 2

parts

parts of the hands of the domeftics employed
in milking, and fometimes on the wrifts, which
quickly run on to fuppuration, firft affuming
the appearance of fmall vefications, produced
by a burn. Moft commonly they appear about
the joints of the fingers, and at their extremities; but whatever parts are affected, if the
fituation will admit, thefe fuperficial fuppura-
tions put on a circular form, with their edges
more elevated than their centre, and of a colour
diftantly approaching to blue. Abforption
takes place, and tumours appear in each axilla.
The fyftem becomes affected — the pulfe is
quickened; and fhiverings, with general laffi-
tude and pains about the loins and limbs, with
vomiting, come on. The head is painful, and
the patient is now and then even affected with
delirium. Thefe fymptoms, varying in their
degree of violence, generally continue from
one day to three or four, leaving ulcerated
fores

fores about the hands, which, from the fenfi-
bility of the parts, are very troublefome, and
commonly heal flowly, frequently becoming
phagedenic, like thofe from whence they
fprung."

" Thus the difeafe makes its progrefs from
the horfe to the nipple of the cow, and from
the cow to the human fubject."

Since no fatal effects have ever been known
to arife from the Cow-pox, even when im-
preffed in the moft unfavourable manner; and
fince this difeafe appears from numerous inftances to leave the conftitution in a ftate of
perfect fecurity from the infection of the
Small-pox, Dr. Jenner infers, that the employ-
ment of the matter of Cow-pox would be
preferable to that of the Small-pox, for the
purpofe of inoculation. In confirmation of his
opinion, it may be obferved, that he relates
the cafes of feven or eight perfons whom he
fuccefs-

succefsfully inoculated with this new antidote to the variolous poifon.

Poffeffed of the above information, I con-fefs I became very anxious to try the effect of inoculating the matter of this fingular difeafe; and as trials could be made not only with fafety, but alfo with the profpect of advantage, I conceived it to be a duty that I owed to the public in my official fituation at the Inoculation Hofpital, to embrace the firft opportunity of carrying the plan into exe-cution.

Unfortunately, however, at the time Dr. Jenner's publication appeared, no Cow-pox matter could be procured, for the difeafe had then become extinct; nor was it expected to return till the fpring, the period at which it ufually affects the cows. But conceiving that the diftemper might be produced by inoculating the nipples of cows with the matter of the

greafe

greafe of horfes, in conformity with the opinion above-ftated, I proceeded to try whether the Cow-pox could be actually excited in this manner.

Numerous experiments were accordingly made upon different cows, with the matter of greafe, taken in the various ftages of that difeafe, but without producing the defired effect: my friend, Mr. Coleman, the ingenious Profeffor at the Veterinary College, likewife made fimilar trials, which proved equally unfuccefsful.* Neither were inoculations with this matter, nor with feveral other morbid fecretions in the horfe, productive of any effects upon the human fubject.

I am aware, that the experiments I allude to, may, by fome, not be deemed wholly con-

* Mr. Coleman caufed one of his cows to be inoculated in its teats with Cow-pox matter, and with that taken from a variolous puftule, without effect; but the former matter, after being regenerated by the human fubject, produced the difeafe in the cow.

clufive,

clusive, from a supposition that the peculiar predisposition of the cows, necessary to render the inoculations efficient, might not exist at the time the matter was applied to their nipples. But I have also other reasons for believing that the Cow-pox does not originate from any disease of the horse. In the first place, the affirmative opinion is confessedly gratuitous: a horse, at a certain season of the year, becomes affected with the grease, and the cows about the same time are affected with Cow-pox; and from this coincidence the two diseases have been considered as cause and effect. Yet is it not equally probable, that the same temporary causes which produce a certain disorder in one animal, may so operate upon another animal of a different genus as to excite another disorder? Therefore, though the Cow-pox may break out among the cows at the time that the grease affects the

horses,

horfes kept on the fame farm, yet the confe-
cutive appearance of thefe difeafes, affords no
proof of their connexion: while on the other
hand I can adduce inftances, in which the
former difeafe has broke out under fuch circumftances as render it highly improbable, if
not impoffible, that it fhould have been caufed
by the latter.*

But though Dr. Jenner feems to have been
mifled with refpect to the origin of the Cow-
pox, ftill his facts and obfervations concerning
its effects upon mankind are not the lefs valid
and important; nor did I feel the lefs defirous
to try how far they would be invalidated or
confirmed by a more enlarged experience than
he had the opportunity of acquiring.

Towards the latter end of January laft I
was informed that the Cow-pox had appeared

* Thofe who wifh for further information on this fubject, may
confult Mr. Simmons's *Experiments*, and Dr. Pearfon's *Inquiry*,
p. 83. & 84.

among

among feveral of the milch cows kept in Gray's-Inn-Lane, and upon examination of thefe, three or four were difcovered to be affected with puftular fores upon their teats and udder. Thefe puftules correfponded in their appearance with the reprefentation and defcription of the genuine Cow-pox, as given by Dr. Jenner; I fhould not, however, call the furrounding inflammation eryfipelatous; it was evidently an indurated tumefaction of the fkin. The number of cows kept at this place was at the time about two hundred, and about four-fifths of them were eventually infected.* The hands of three or four perfons became fore in confequence of milking the cows thus affected; and one of them, (Sarah Rice) exhibited fo perfect a fpecimen of the difeafe, that I could entertain no doubt of its being the true and not the fpurious Cow-pox.

* Thofe cows which were not in milk efcaped the difeafe.

Several

Several gentlemen, who I knew would be highly gratified by feeing the difeafe as it appeared upon this girl's arm, were invited to meet me at the Cow-houfe on the following day, when Lord Somerville, Sir Jofeph Banks, Sir Wm. Watfon, Drs. Simmons, Pearfon, Willan, and others, attended. This was on the 24th of January laft, and Sarah Rice had then been affected five days. The appearance of the difeafe upon this girl's hand and arm very much refembled the reprefentation of it given in the firft plate of Dr. Jenner's pamphlet. At firft a fmall tumour, or circular vefication appeared between her fingers; next day fhe difcovered three more like the firft, viz. one upon her finger, another at the wrift, and alfo one upon the middle of her fore-arm. The two firft never became larger, and exactly refembled the veficle upon the finger in the plate alluded to; that at the wrift was now about

one-

one-third of an inch in diameter, and the
other upon her arm was ftill larger : they were
both of a circular form, not depreffed at the
centre, and had a fimple inflammatory border. The pellicle of both thefe tumours, but
more efpecially of the larger, had at this
time acquired a blue colour, which was
deepeft about the centre. This bluenefs had
come on during the laft twenty-four hours;
for I had feen the tumours the preceding day,
when this coloured tinge could fcarcely be
perceived, and that too only in the largeft ;
at that time alfo it contained a colourlefs fluid,
but now its contents appeared brownifh. The
girl now perceived an uneafinefs at the axilla;
and I afterwards learned that this fymptom
was followed by a flight head-ach. None of
the tumours were painful, and they all gradually went off without producing ulceration.

Sarah Rice had undergone the Small-pox
when

when a child; and the only reafon why fhe was more affected by milking the difeafed cows than the other milkers were, was, that her hands and arms were more red, fwollen, and difpofed to chap than theirs; though it does not appear that there were any abrafions of the cuticle of thofe parts of the fkin which were infected by the Cow-pox.

Before relating the cafes of inoculation with the matter of Cow-pox, I have judged it proper in the firft place briefly to ftate what are the local effects produced by inoculating variolous matter, fo that the progrefs of the infection in both cafes may be compared, and the fubject of inoculation at large, be better underftood.

In cafes wherein inoculation of the Small-pox proves effectual, a fmall particle of variolous matter being applied by a fuperficial puncture of the fkin, ufually produces in the

courfe

courfe of three or four days, or fooner, a
little elevation of the punctured part, difcover-
able by the touch, and a red fpeck diftin-
guifhable by the eye. From this time the
rednefs advances in a circular form, more or
lefs rapidly, according to the conftitutional
circumftances of the patient; and the firft
effect of this fuperficial inflammation is the
formation of a veficle upon its centre, which
ufually appears between the fourth and feventh day after the inoculation. The extent
of this veficle is generally found to bear
fome proportion to the intenfity of the inflammation: and contains a limpid fluid, by
the abforption of which, the Small-pox is
produced. The veficle foon burfts, and the
central part of the puncture becomes depreffed,
and often of a dark hue; which appearances,
together with the marginal inflammation,
continue to increafe till the eruptive fymptoms

toms fubfide, when the edges of the depreffed part begin to fwell with a purulent fluid, and the inflammation gradually recedes.

Thus it appears that the variolous matter, firft inferted by the punɗure, like that of other morbid poifons, is not capable of being immediately abforbed, but lodges in the fkin, and there excites an inflammatory procefs, by which a new matter, producing the difeafe, is generated.* It would feem alfo that this pro-cefs is carried to a greater or lefs extent in different perfons before the matter enters the abforbents, owing probably to the greater or lefs aptitude in thefe veffels to receive it. Hence we find the local inflammation in fome cafes confiderably advanced before the fyftem becomes affeɗed; while in others the eruptive

* In the fecond Volume of the *Hiftory of Inoculation,* (now nearly ready for the prefs) I have endeavoured to fhow that the general greater mildnefs of the inoculated than the cafual Small-pox, depends upon this circumftance.

fymptoms

symptoms supervene, when it appears to have made but very little progress, and therefore though the eighth day after the inoculation proves the usual period at which the patient feels indisposed, yet this frequently happens much sooner or later, and the progress of the Cow-pox infection will be found to take the same latitude.

Monday, January 21, 1799, I took the matter of Cow-pox, in a purulent state, from the teats of a cow, with which I immediately inoculated seven persons by a single puncture, in the arm of each, or rather by scratching the skin with the point of the lancet, till the instrument became tinged with blood.

FIRST CASE.

Mary Payne, a child two years and an half old, of a strong robust constitution. 3d day.

The

the inoculated part was evidently elevated, and
flightly inflamed—6th day the local tumour
extended to about one-third of an inch in diameter, and was nearly of a circular form with
its edges more elevated than the centre, and
with the furrounding inflammation not greater
than is ufual in cafes of inoculated Small-pox:
the veficle upon the middle of the tumour was
now very large, and diftended with a limpid
fluid; fome of which I took upon a lancet,
and with it inoculated another perfon, John
Talley. She appeared dull and drowfy; and
her pulfe was quicker than ufual. She had
no appetite for food, and had been very
thirfty fince yefterday. 8th day. The rednefs furrounding the tumour feems retiring;
and the thirft and other febrile fymptoms are
much abated; but fhe ftill appears liftlefs and
fomewhat indifpofed. 11th day. She is perfectly free from complaint: the inoculated part

c   is

is fcabbing, but furrounded with a hard tumefaction, of a bright red colour. She was this
day inoculated with variolous matter. 15th
day. She has no ailment. The variolous
inoculation produced confiderable inflammation, which gradually difappeared after the
fifth day.

————

SECOND CASE.

Elizabeth Payne, aged four months, in appearance weak, and fomewhat emaciated.
The progrefs of the infection on this child's
arm was very much like that of her fifter's
juft mentioned; but the vefication feemed
rather more extenfive, and the furrounding
inflammation lefs. The fixth day after inoculation, her mother informed me that the child
had been very unwell the preceding night with
what

what were called inward convulfions, and had vomited two or three times. On examination, the heat of her fkin, and the frequency of her pulfe, indicated the prefence of fome degree of fever. 8th day. I learned that the febrile ftate had continued, more or lefs, till this morning; nor was it then wholly gone off. The inoculated part, I judged from its appearance, had not entirely ceafed from difordering the conftitution. 11th day. The rednefs of the tumour is fubfiding, and its general appearance refembles the effects of inoculation with variolous matter when the eruption is completed, and the maturation proceeding favourably. The patient's mother now thinks her as well as ufual. She was this day inoculated with variolous matter. 13th day. She manifefts no figns of indifpofition. The rednefs about the tumour is gone off, and the matter is forming a fcab. The fecond inoculation

produces

produces no effect. 15th day. She is now very well; but her mother says she was seized with inward convulsions yesterday, and was extremely ill afterward for two hours: this, however, cannot be justly ascribed to inoculation, as the part in which the Cow-pox matter was inserted is now covered with a dry scab, not attended with inflammation; and the variolous matter produced no redness whatever. She was this day brought to a man labouring under the casual Small-pox, and kissed by him, in order more fully to try if she was secure from the infection of the Small-pox. Her sister, Mary Payne, was also subjected to the same test, but neither of them have since taken the disease.

THIRD

THIRD CASE.

Thomas Buckland, a ſtrong child, four months old.—The progreſs of the infection on this boy's arm was even more regular, and produced appearances more analogous to thoſe of the inoculated Small-pox than in the caſe of Mary Payne. The veſicle on the inoculated part formed on the third day, and the ſurrounding inflammation never became phlegmonous, nor was attended with any hardneſs of the integuments. 7th day. In the evening, he was diſcovered to be feveriſh and reſtleſs, when two puſtules, exactly reſembling thoſe of the Small-pox, appeared near to the inoculated part. The following day he ſtill continued indiſpoſed, and the cutaneous inflammation had that peculiar irritable or angry aſpect which is obſervable on the acceſſion of the eruptive ſymptoms in caſes of inoculation

with

with variolous matter. 10th day. The fuppuration was more extended, and the efflorefcence immediately encompaffing it, had
nearly difappeared, leaving its outer border
more ftrongly marked than the inner; a circumftance of the moft favourable import in
inoculation. The two puftules upon his arm
were more advanced, and feveral others were
now vifible upon different parts of his body:
his ankles and feet were befet with a rafh
like the fcarlatina. He is ftill feverifh, and
his mother reports, that laft night he vomited.
11th day. The forenefs of his arm, and the
fever had ceafed. Nine diftinct puftules were
now difcovered upon his body and limbs,
fomewhat fmaller than variolous puftules: from
one of thefe I obtained an ichorous matter,
and with it inoculated Sarah Price. 13th day.
The febrile fymptoms returned yefterday, nor
is he wholly free from them to-day. Nine
additional

additional puſtules have appeared: no inflammation remains at the inoculated part, and
the matter it contains begins to dry. 15th
day. He is free from diforder: fix puſtules
more have appeared, making in the whole
twenty-four, fome of them maturate at the
apex, but they moſtly die away without proceeding to fuppuration. He was this day expofed to the effluvia of the cafual Small-pox,
in the fame manner as the two Paynes.

FOURTH CASE.

Richard Payne, a healthy boy, ten years
old. The inoculated part was not fenfibly
elevated nor inflamed, till the fourth day.
7th day. The tumour had fpread-confider-
ably, and the vefication upon it was very evident. He felt a fenfation of itching in the
part; and the next day complained of a pain
in

in the axilla, which continued two days. 10th day. The centre of the tumour became depreffed, its edges elevated, and furrounded by a deep-coloured inflammatory border. The central part of the tumour was now affuming externally a brown colour, and in a few days afterwards it formed a dark fcab. Though confiderable tumefaction, with hardnefs and rednefs, remained at the inoculated part feveral days, yet no ulceration enfued. 15th day. Five puftules appeared, refembling thofe in Buckland. This boy was twice inoculated with variolous matter during the progrefs of the Cow-pox infection, and expofed to patients under the Small-pox the whole time, without being infected by it; and the only complaint arifing from the Cow-pox was the pain in his arm-pit.

FIFTH

FIFTH CASE.

Matthew Redding, fixteen years old. 3d day. The infertion of the matter did not appear to have produced any inflammation or hardnefs in the part : he was therefore inoculated with variolous matter, at the diftance of two inches from the part in which the Cowpox matter was inferted. Next day, a little rednefs could be difcovered at the firft puncture, and from this time both inoculations proceeded very regularly, but flowly, fo that on the feventh day they appeared to be inflamed in an equal degree, the extent of the inflammation not exceeding the tenth of an inch in diameter. 8th day.* He has pain in the axilla.

* Here, as well as in the fubfequent cafes, where the patient was twice inoculated on different days, I date the time from the firft inoculation.

10th day.

10th day. Both tumours are approaching to fuppuration. They are of the fame form, and attended with an equal degree of efflorefcence. 11th day. He complains of headach: the red tinge now extends in a circular form, and includes both tumours. 13th day. There appears more tenfion and pain at the variolous tumour than at the other, but the latter tumour is more prominent. 15th day. Both tumours began to dry, and no inconvenience followed. This boy made no other complaint, during the procefs of infection, than of uneafinefs in the axilla, followed by a flight head-ach, of very fhort duration: however, on the 17th day, four fmall puftules appeared, viz. one upon his nofe, one upon his thigh, and two on his head; none of which fuppurated. This cafe ftrikingly refembles that of Richard Payne, in which the puftules did not appear till the arm fcabbed.

SIXTH

SIXTH CASE.

Jane Collingridge, a healthy active girl, feventeen years of age. 3d day. The inoculated part began to be elevated and inflamed. 5th day. It was veficated, and attended with itching. She was now inoculated with variolous matter in the right arm, the former inoculation having been in the left. 8th day. The whole tumour is much increafed in all dimenfions; its form is perfectly circular, and it appears of a lemon-coloured tint. She now complains of a ftiffnefs acrofs her arms, and of a pain in the left axilla: the puncture in the right arm begins to be elevated and inflamed. 11th day. She complains of headach, and pain about the loins: the tumour produced by the Cow-pox matter is now more inflamed at the margin, which is befet with minute confluent puftules: the variolous tu-

mour

mour is alſo advanced to a ſtate of veſication; and ſhe reports, that laſt night both
axillæ were painful. 12th day. She continues
indiſpoſed : the tumour is ſurrounded by an
extenſive efflorescence : the variolous tumour is of a deeper red colour. 13th day.
The Cow-pox tumour is ſubſiding, and forming a ſcab : that of the Small-pox is efflor-
eſcent : her head-ach continues : pain in the
right axilla : ſeveral puſtules appear. 15th
day. There are ſmall puſtules round the edges
of the variolous tumour : more puſtules
appear ſcattered over the face, body, and
limbs. 17th day. The ſcab over the Cow-pox
tumour is completely formed ; at its edges,
however, a fluid is ſtill viſible : the variolous
tumour is in a ſtate of ſuppuration : ſhe complains of a ſore throat : the number of puſtules
is now from one to two hundred, in no reſpect
differing from variolous puſtules of the mild
ſort.

fort. From this time both the tumours gradually healed, and the puftules dried at the
ufual time.

SEVENTH CASE.

Ann Pink, a tall girl, of a brown fallow
complexion, aged fifteen years. This girl was
inoculated with variolous matter, on the fifth
day, in the fame manner as Collingridge, and
both tumours proceeded to maturation, though
more flowly than in that cafe. Neither of the
tumours began to fcab till the feventeenth day,
when they refembled each other fo perfectly,
that the one could not eafily be diftinguifhed
from the other. She had no pain in either
axilla, nor made any complaint during the
whole progrefs of the infection, neither did
one puftule appear upon her.

The only other perfons whom I firft inoculated

lated with the matter of Cow-pox, and on the
fifth day afterwards with variolous matter,
were William Harris, William Bunker, and
James Crouch.

——————

EIGHTH CASE.

William Harris, twenty-one years of age,
of a tall and flender make, and of a delicate
conftitution, was inoculated January 24, with
the matter of Cow-pox, taken from the arm
of Sarah Rice, who received the difeafe by
milking the cows. 3d day. The inoculated
part was evidently elevated and inflamed.
5th day. It advanced to vefication, and a fenfation of itching was perceived in the part :
he was this day inoculated was variolous
matter. 9th day. The tumour of the firft
inoculation prefents prominent callous edges,
with but very little rednefs; its centre is
depreffed, and contains a lymphatic fluid : he
perceives

perceives a tendernefs in the axilla: the variolous tumour is confiderably inflamed and veficated, and itches more than the other. Next
day a pain was perceived in the axilla of the
arm in which the variolous matter was inferted, as well as in the other. 12th day.
rednefs of the Cow-pox tumour is going off;
but that of the variolous ftill fpreads with
an irregular margin. 14th day. Several
puftules appear. The Cow-pox tumour is
now dry at the centre, but its furrounding
edges appear of a blueifh tinge, and ftill
abound with ichorous matter. The variolous tumour is much inflamed, and befet with
confluent puftules at its edges: its centre is depreffed, and of a dark hue. 19th day. The
Cow-pox tumour has formed into a dry fcab,
with a finely polifhed furface, and of a ma-
hogany-brown colour: the variolous tumour
is in a purulent ftate, with an extenfive inflammation

flammation at the margin: the puftules are about 300 in number, very large, and all in a ftate of maturation. From this time all the effects of inoculation went off gradually: he never complained of head-ach, nor of any febrile fymptom during the whole progrefs of the difeafe.

———

NINTH CASE.

Wm. Bunker, a ftrong healthy boy, fifteen years of age, was inoculated, in his left arm, on the fame day, and with matter from the fame perfon as Harris. 3d day. The inoculated part was elevated and reddened. 5th day. The inflammation was much increafed: he was now inoculated in his right arm with va-riolous matter. 8th day. The tumour upon his left arm is much elevated, and the vefica-tion confiderable fince the fixth day: he now

complains

complains of pain in the axilla, and of head-
ach. The puftule on the right arm advances
very flowly. 10th day. The pain in the
axilla and the head-ach continue. The tumour of the left arm begins to fcab in
the centre, and is furrounded with a red
tinge of confiderable extent. The tumour
on the right arm now alfo prefents a red tinge
of a fimilar appearance, but not of half the
extent: its centre is in a ftate of vefication,
and its edges ftudded with fmall puftules: his
head-ach is not entirely gone off. 12th day.
The red tinge furrounding the tumour on the
left arm has difappeared, except a narrow
ring at its outer ambit: the tumour on the
right arm is depreffed at the centre, where it
is alfo of a livid colour; its edges are hard
and inflamed: he now difcovers two or three
puftules upon his body. 17th day. The
matter of both tumours is almoft wholly

E   formed

formed into a dry incruftation: no more puftules have appeared : one upon his hip has
maturated. 20th day. Both tumours are
perfectly fcabbed; that upon his left arm
appears browner and fmoother than the other.

———————

TENTH CASE.

James Crouch, feven years old, inoculated
on the fame day as the laft patient with matter taken from the fame girl, and with variolous matter five days afterward. 5th day.
The inoculated part was confiderably elevated
and inflamed. 9th day. The Cow-pox tumour is much advanced: the pellicle filled
with ichor: the marginal inflammation not
confiderable: the variolous puncture now dif-
plays a fmall red fpeck, which begins to fpread.
11th day. The Cow-pox tumour exhibits
an extenfive efflorefcence, or red ftain, upon

the

the furrounding fkin, and its centre begins to dry: the variolous tumour is fpreading a little, and in a ftate of vefication. 14th day. Pain in the axilla is now produced by the Cow-pox tumour, which is drying at the centre: the variolous tumour is now efflor-efcent, but not to half the extent of the other. From this time the tumours quickly healed, no eruption took place, and no farther incon-venience was experienced.

ELEVENTH and TWELFTH CASE.

Thomas Fox, aged twenty-five, and John Dennis, twenty-three years of age, both ftrong men, and accuftomed to hard labour, were inoculated on the 22d of January, with va-riolous matter, and on the following day with Cow-pox matter, taken from the arm of Sarah

E 2 Rice,

Rice. In both these cases, the first inoculation was performed by two punctures at the distance of two inches from each other, and the latter by one puncture at the same distance from the two former. The local effects and appearances of the inoculation were very similar in both these men : the Cow-pox tumours seemed to advance equally with those of the variolous, and bore a strong resemblance to them; the former, however, were more elevated and circumscribed : for about the ninth day the variolous tumours became angulated or ragged at the margin, which was not so conspicuous in the others, though both had small confluent pustules at their margins. Those of the Cow-pox also sooner healed, and formed a smoother scab. The eruptive fever came on about the eighth day with Dennis, but not till the tenth with Fox : the former had more than 300 pustules, and the

latter

latter about 100; all of which were in every refpect fimilar to variolous puftules.

THIRTEENTH and FOURTEENTH CASE.

John Talley, fourteen, and Thomas Brown, fifteen years old, were, January 25th, inoculated with variolous matter in the left arm, and the following day they were both inoculated in the right arm with the matter of Cow-pox, taken from the arms of Mary and Elizabeth Payne, (fee cafes firft and fecond) The progrefs of both the infections on the arms of thefe boys was perfectly regular and equal throughout. On the 7th day all the tumours were confiderably inflamed, and in a ftate of vefication, attended with itching. Brown alfo at this time complained of a pain in each axilla; but with Talley the pain was confined

fined to the left till the next day, when both arm-pits were affected. 10th day. They both complained of head-ach, and of pains about the loins : thefe, however, were very flight, and no further indifpofition enfued. On the evening of the 12th day fome puftules appeared upon Brown, but upon Talley they did not appear till the 14th day : the former had in all about thirty, and the latter only fix, all of which were apparently variolous. The Cowpox tumours were more elevated at the edges, and lefs depreffed at the centre, after the 9th day, than thofe of the variolous ; and they eventually formed a fmoother and browner fcab, as in the cafe of Fox and Dennis.

January 30th—William Mundy, Elizabeth George, and Sarah Butcher, were inoculated by two punctures with the matter of Cowpox, taken from the arm of Collingridge. (Cafe 6th).

FIFTEENTH

FIFTEENTH CASE.

William Mundy, a ftrong labouring man, aged twenty-five years, was inoculated as above defcribed by two punctures in his left arm. The local infection of both punctures advanced, and the inflammation and its effects proceeded rapidly, fo that on the 8th day he complained of uneafinefs in his axilla, and of pain in the head and loins, which continued about two days: the tumours were then confiderably elevated, and their margins much inflamed. 13th day. They were furrounded with an extenfive rednefs, in the form of an halo, and beginning to fcab at the centre: the edges continued circular, well defined, and elevated. 14th day. Several puftules appeared upon his neck and back, but difappeared in two or three days without fuppurating. He was this day inoculated with variolous mat-

ter

ter, but it produced no other effect than a little rednefs, of two or three days duration.

––––––––––

SIXTEENTH CASE.

Elizabeth George, a ftrong woman, twenty-five years old, was inoculated in the fame manner, and on the day above mentioned, with Cow-pox matter taken from the fame perfon. The punctures quickly rofe, but the inflammation was inconfiderable till the fixth day, when vefication and itching commenced. 9th day. Has no pain in the axilla, but complains of head-ach and pain in the loins. 11th day. Her pains continue; pulfe quick; the central pellicle of the tumours is extending, and replete with a watery humour; the margins fwollen, and red. 13th day. The fame appearances continue. 15th day. The fymptoms are abated : fays fhe has no

other

other complaint than a giddinefs of the head:
the inflammation at the margins of the tumours is greatly abated: the matter in the
centre is beginning to dry: fome puftules appear on her face. 16th day. She makes no
complaint: more puftules fhew themfelves:
the tumours appear circular, with the centre
equally elevated as the edges, and exhibiting
an uniform fmooth furface, which is becoming hard. 18th day. More puftules have appeared: the tumours are fcabbing, and the
furrounding rednefs is almoft wholly gone.
20th day. Her face is fwelled; the puftules
are very fore, and in a purulent ftate; their
number is 530, and two in the throat are a
little troublefome. 25th day. The puftules
in a ftate of defquamation. She was now
inoculated with variolous matter, which produced no effect. The fcabs at the inoculated
parts were of that brown fmooth kind peculiar to the Cow-pox.

F SEVEN-

SEVENTEENTH CASE.

Sarah Butcher, a healthy little girl, thirteen years old, was inoculated with the matter of Cow-pox, at the fame time and in the fame manner as above mentioned. 6th day. The tumours were much elevated: the inflammation inconfiderable: the vefication fully formed, and attended with itching. 9th day. There was a flight efflorefcence around the tumours: uneafinefs in the axilla: head-ach: pain in the loins. 11th day. Suppuration at the inner edges of the tumours: rednefs at the outer edge very extenfive. 14th day. Tumours fcabbing: no eruption: complains of pain in her bowels, and diarrhœa. 16th day. No complaint: central part of the tumours fcabbed: inflammation ftill furrounding the edges. She was inoculated this day with variolous matter. 18th day. The rednefs gone

off,

off, leaving a red tinge at its outer margin. The variolous inoculation produced a little rednefs, which difappeared in two days.

January 31ft. Thomas Wife, aged fourteen, and Sarah Price, aged thirteen years, were inoculated with the matter of Cow-pox, taken from Matthew Redding, and at the fame time with variolous matter; but the effects of the latter inoculations were the following day prevented by applying the concentrated acid of vitriol to the punctures.

EIGHTEENTH CASE.

Thomas Wife, above-mentioned. 5th day. The inoculated part was confiderably inflamed and veficated. 8th day. The tumour advances with much marginal rednefs; and a pain in the axilla is perceived. 12th day. Pain in the axilla continued two days: he has had no

F 2   other

other complaint: the centre of the tumour is forming a ſcab, but is ſurrounded with an appearance like the areola papillæ: two puſtules were diſcovered upon his body this day, and two more appeared on the 15th day, but none of them became purulent: the tumour upon his arm had at that time formed a hard ſmooth ſcab.

NINETEENTH CASE.

Sarah Price, inoculated as above ſtated, in her left arm. On the ſame day was inſerted in her right arm Cow-pox matter, taken from a puſtule from Buckland. 5th day. There was a redneſs and elevation at the two punctures each arm, but, in conſequence of the cauſtic effects of the vitriolic acid, none at the variolous puncture. 8th day. Both tumours were advanced: veſication, and a conſiderable degree of inflammation, eſpecially in that on

the

the left arm. She now complains of *rigor*, and of a pain in the left axilla. Thefe fymptoms, together with a head-ach, continued two days. 13th day. No complaint: both tumours fubfiding: three fmall puftules have appeared upon her face and neck, and two days afterwards three others, none of which fuppurated. This girl, as well as Thomas Wife, was conftantly expofed to the Small-pox during the progrefs of their inoculation,

---

TWENTIETH CASE.

Thomas Dorfet, inoculated February 1ft with the matter of Cow-pox, taken from the arm of Jane Collingridge, (fee cafe 6th). 7th day. The inoculated part was much elevated, and in a ftate of vefication, attended with the ufual degree of rednefs. 11th day. Laft night he perceived an uneafinefs in his axilla,

axilla, and he now complains of pain about his loins: the tumour encircled by an extensive efflorescence. 13th day. The tumour scabbing at the centre: he was inoculated this day with variolous matter. The variolous inoculation produced no effect. About the 12th day this man had four or five pustular appearances, which he called pocks; but they seemed to me more like common pimples than variolous pustules.

TWENTY-FIRST CASE.

John Keys, twenty-five years old, inoculated February 4, with matter of Cow-pox taken from the arm of James Crouch. On the fourth day the inoculated part was considerably inflamed, and affected with a sensation of itching; but from this time the redness gradually disappeared, and was entirely gone on the ninth day, when he was

inoculated

inoculated with variolous matter in both arms, but without effect. On the tenth day, however, he complained of pain in his head and loins, with which he was affected three days, but no eruption enfued.

TWENTY-SECOND CASE.

Edward Turner, a ftrong man, twenty-four years of age, inoculated by two punctures with the matter of Cow-pox taken from the arm of James Crouch (Cafe 10th) Feb. 5th. 7th day. The tumours were much advanced, in a ftate of open vefication, and attended with itching. 12th day. They began to dry in the centre, but the margins were of a dark red colour, and ftudded with minute veficulæ: he now complains of pain in the axilla, ftiffnefs of his neck, and pain in the loins. 14th day. Head-ach and pain in the loins continue:

tinue: the inner edges of the tumours are diſtended with an ichorous fluid. 16th day. Complains of head-ach, and fore throat: next day about 100 puſtules appeared, many of which were very ſmall. 19th day. He has no complaint: the number of the puſtules now amounts to about 220: all of them afterwards ſuppurated. On the 23d day he was inoculated with the variolous matter, which produced no effect.

TWENTY-THIRD CASE.

Hannah Morgan, a ſtrong child, one year old, was inoculated with the matter of Cow-pox taken from the arm of James Crouch, Feb. 5. 5th day. The inoculated part is much elevated and inflamed. 7th day. The tumour contains ichor, and the redneſs and elevation are greatly increaſed: yeſterday ſhe became feveriſh, and laſt night was ſick and vomited: her

her fkin at this time is hotter than ufual. 14th day. The febrile fymptoms continued, and at times were very fevere, till the eleventh day, fince which time they have not returned: no puftules have appeared, and the tumour is now fcabbing. She was afterwards inoculated with variolous matter, but it only produced a tranfient rednefs in the part.

TWENTY-FOURTH CASE.

Jane Weft, twenty-one years of age, was inoculated Feb. 6th with the matter of Cow-pox taken from the arm of Sarah Butcher. 7th day. The inoculated part was confider-ably elevated and inflamed; the vefication was alfo extenfive, and attended with itching. 9th day. She complained of head-ach, and next day of a pain in the axilla, and upon her fhoulder, attended with rigors and fhiver-

G   ing;

ing: the border of the tumour appeared of a deep red, and its inner edges contained an ichorous matter. 13th day. Yesterday an efflorescence appeared round the tumour. She complains of a sore throat, and says she has a pain acrofs her cheft. 15th day. Two puftules have appeared upon her fide : the tumour begins to dry. She makes no complaint. 17th day. Twenty puftules appeared, all of which fuppurated. 23d day. The variolous inoculation produced no inflammation.

TWENTY-FIFTH CASE.

Ann Bumpus, aged twenty years, was inoculated Feb. 6, with the matter of Cow-pox, taken from the arm of Sarah Butcher. The appearances of the inoculated part in this girl's arm, corresponded in every respect with those ftated in Weft's cafe. 8th day. She

She complained of head-ach. 10th day. Pain of the head and loins; fhiverings. 11th day. Two or three puftules appear upon her face. 13th day. Pains continue; more puftules appear. 15th day. No complaint: the puftules were counted and found to be 310, refembling thofe of the Small-pox. 17th day. Complains of fore throat. 19th day. Puftules drying. 22d day. Inoculated with the matter of Small-pox, but no inflammation was produced by it.

TWENTY-SIXTH CASE.

Thomas Slade, twenty years of age, was inoculated with the matter of Cow-pox, taken from the arm of William Mundy, Feb. 6. On the eighth day the inoculated part was much elevated, and in an advanced ftate of veication. He complained of head-ach, and pain

in

in the axilla; and on the next day of a pain in the loins. 11th day. Pains abated, three or four puftules appear; the tumour is bordered with fmall confluent veficles. 14th day. No complaints; tumour beginning to fcab. 19th day. The centre of the tumour formed a brown hard fcab. The puftules do not fuppurate, and are receding. 22d day. He was inoculated with the matter of Small-pox, which produced a rednefs for two or three days, and afterwards gradually difappeared.

TWENTY-SEVENTH CASE.

Frances Jewel, a healthy young woman, twenty years of age, who had undergone the Small-pox by inoculation when a child, was inoculated with the matter of Cow-pox taken from the arm of Sarah Butcher, Feb. 5. The inoculated part advanced into a tumour equal

in

in extent and duration to that in the cafe laft mentioned: on the 9th day, head-ach and pain of the loins came on, and continued two or three days. The tumour began to fcab on the 13th day, but no puftules appeared. She was afterwards inoculated with variolous matter, and alfo with that of the Cow-pox, neither of which produced any inflammation.

TWENTY-EIGHTH CASE.

Charlotte Fifk, four months old, was, on February the 13th, inoculated with the matter of Cow-pox, taken from the arm of Frances Jewel. In this child the local difeafe proceeded very regularly. She became indifpofed on the eighth day, and continued feverifh for three or four days, when about forty puftules appeared; but the greateft part of thefe puftules did not proceed to fuppuration. The mother

of

of this child laboured under the natural Small-
pox, and was covered with puftules in a purulent ftate at the time her child was inoculated;
yet the infant was fuckled by her during the
whole courfe of the difeafe, and was frequently
feen befmeared with variolous pus. Whence
it would appear, that the vaccine infection
not only prevents but actually fuperfedes the
cafual Small-pox.

————

TWENTY-NINTH CASE.

James Tarrent, nineteen years old, was, on
the 16th of February, inoculated with the
matter of Cow-pox, taken from a puftule
upon Eliz. George. In this cafe the inflammation at the inoculated part proceeded very
rapidly, and was more extenfive than ufual on
the fixth day; but from this time it began to
recede, and was entirely gone on the tenth day,
only a fmall dry fcab at the puncture being left.

He

He was now inoculated with variolous matter, which did not produce any inflammation whatever. I confider this man as one of the few whofe conftitutions cannot be affected either by the virus of the Cow-pox, or the Small-pox. It is true he complained of head-ach about the ninth day, but I fhould not be difpofed to attribute this fymptom to the inoculation.

THIRTIETH CASE.

William Hull, aged eleven years, was, on the 8th of February, inoculated with the matter of Cow-pox, taken from the arm of Sarah Butcher. 7th day. The tumour at the inoculated part is advanced in the ufual manner, and he this day complains of head-ach. 10th day. His head-ach and pain in the loins continue; and feveral puftules now appear upon him. 12th day. The pains are gone off, and

more

more puſtules have appeared. 15th day. The puſtules amount to about 200. They vary much in ſize, and are proceeding to maturation. 18th day. He was inoculated with variolous matter, which produced no effect.

THIRTY-FIRST & THIRTY-SECOND CASE.

February 8th, Hannah Hull, aged thirteen years, and Sarah Hull, eight years old, were inoculated with the matter of Cow-pox taken from Sarah Butcher.

Theſe two ſiſters had the diſeaſe rather more favourably than their brother Wm. Hull, for the inoculated part was in both ſurrounded by an effloreſcence on the 11th day, and the number of puſtules upon the two was not equal to that of their brother's, nor were the eruptive ſymptoms of half the duration of his. On the 20th day they were inoculated for the Small-pox, but no diſeaſe enſued.

THIRTY-

THIRTY-THIRD CASE.

George Reed, aged fifteen years, was inoculated with the matter of Cow-pox taken from the arm of F. Jewel, February 14th. The inoculated part tumified in the ufual manner: he complained of head-ach on the eighth day, and this fymptom continued with occafional intermiffions till the 13th day. Some puftules began to appear about the 11th, and the eruption was completed on the 14th day. They were in number about 70, fome of which were very fmall, but they all maturated in a favourable manner. He was afterwards inoculated with variolous matter, which formed a puftular appearance; but no diforder was produced.

———

Frances Pedder, Amelia Hoole, George Hickland, and Elizabeth Morton, were inoculated on February 13th and 14th with Cow-pox matter taken from the arm of Sarah Price, who was inoculated from a puftule on Buckland, (fee cafe 3d).

THIRTY-FOURTH CASE.

Frances Pedder, a child eleven months old. The inoculated part was gradually elevated and inflamed. 8th day. The eruptive fymptoms fupervened, and fhe continued feverifh till the 13th day, when feveral puftules appeared. 16th day. The tumour began to fcab, and the number of puftules then upon her was 40, all of which maturated without becoming purulent. She was afterwards inoculated for the Small-pox without effect.

THIRTY-FIFTH CASE.

Amelia Hoole, five months old, was inoculated as above defcribed. The local tumour advanced in the ufual manner. 7th day. She became feverifh, and feveral fmall puftules
appeared

appeared at the border of the tumour. 10th day. She has continued flightly indifpofed fince the laft report, and nine puftules are now vifible upon her body and extremities. 14th day. The puftules amount to 102 in number, and form yellowifh fcabs. 18th day. The inoculated part was perfectly healed: the puftules appeared in a ftate of defquamation. She was at this time inoculated with variolous matter, but without effect.

THIRTY-SIXTH CASE.

George Hickland, fix months old, inoculated from the perfon above mentioned. The eruptive fymptoms in this child were lefs fevere, and of fhorter duration than in the laft cafe. However, the number of puftules which appeared amounted to 300, but only about one-third of them fuppurated. This patient alfo refifted the infection of the Small-pox by inoculation.

H 2   THIRTY-

THIRTY-SEVENTH CASE.

Elizabeth Morton, nine months old, was more feverely difordered than any of the four children inoculated with the matter taken from Sarah Price. The fever continued with fome degree of violence from the 7th to the 15th day, and the number of puftules amounted to 200. On the 20th day fhe was inoculated with variolous matter without effect.

THIRTY-EIGHTH CASE.

L. Davy, aged eleven weeks, was, on Feb. 19th, inoculated with the matter of Cow-pox taken from the arm of Charlotte Fifk. This child had the difeafe very favourably. On the 10th day the tumour was furrounded by an efflorefcence, and her fkin was a little hotter than ufual during that day only. On the 13th day one puftule appeared near to the inoculated part, and two upon her forehead, which

were

were all fhe had. She was afterwards inoculated for the Small-pox without effect.

———

THIRTY-NINTH CASE.

Maria Murrell, aged feven months, was
inoculated with matter taken from the fame
perfon and on the fame day as Davy. 5th
day. The inoculated part was much elevated
and inflamed. On the evening of the 8th day
fhe vomited 10th day. The tumour was
furrounded by a very extenfive efflorefcence,
and fhe became hot and reftlefs. 12th day.
She feemed free from fever, and about twenty
puftules appeared upon her. 14th day. The
inflammation upon the arm was gone off,
and the puftules feemed to be fcabbing. The
fubfequent inoculation of the Small-pox, as
upon the others, produced no effect upon this
patient.

A cow,

A cow, kept by Profeſſor Coleman, at the Veterinary College, was inoculated in its teat with the matter of Cow-pox taken from the arm of James Crouch, which produced the diſeaſe in the cow, (ſee caſe 10th). A man-ſervant, by milking this cow, was alſo affected with an extenſive tumour upon his thumb: this ſoon acquired a livid blue colour, and was attended with a conſiderable degree of fever for ſeveral days, and with a raſh upon his ankles and feet.

With the matter produced in the nipple of this cow were inoculated Martha Streeton, James Smith, and George Meacock.

FORTIETH CASE.

Martha Streeton, aged twenty-two years, was, on the 18th of February, inoculated with the matter above mentioned. The inoculated part tumified in the uſual manner, and on the

9th

9th day fhe complained of head-ach, and afterwards of a pain in the axilla. The head-ach
and pain in the loins continued, but not with
feverity, for five or fix days. Puftules began
to appear on the 12th, and the eruption was
completed on the 16th day, when the number
was about 300. During the maturation of
the puftules, which in no refpect differed from
thofe of the Small-pox, fhe complained of
her throat being fore. On the 19th day this
patient was perfectly well. She was afterwards inoculated for the Small-pox without
effect.

FORTY-FIRST & FORTY-SECOND CASE.

James Smith, fixteen, and George Meacock, thirty years of age, were, on the 19th
of February, inoculated with the fame matter
as that mentioned in the preceding cafe. The
latter of thefe patients had the difeafe nearly

in

in the fame manner as Streeton; but in a greater degree, for Meacock's puftules were more numerous, and the inoculated part did not exhibit a tumour fo well defined and elevated as Streeton's did. Smith's cafe differed widely from both; his arm tumified rapidly, and an erythema or blufh extended from the punéture feveral inches up his arm, and down to his elbow. The eruptive fymptoms began on the 7th, and continued in a flight degree till the 11th day. He had four or five puftules upon his face, and nearly 100 upon his body and limbs, all of which maturated favourably, and the eryfipelatous appearance at the inoculated part foon went off, though no application was employed for that purpofe.

Both the above patients were inoculated with variolous matter, which produced no effeét upon Meacock, but in Smith it was followed by a cutaneous inflammation of feveral days continuance.

Samuel

Samuel Fairbrother, fifteen years old; Richard Calloway, aged nineteen; James Camplin, aged feventeen years; John Turner, eight months old; Joanna Buckley, five months old; and Mary Welch, three months old, were all, on the 21ft and 23d of February, inoculated with the matter of Cow-pox, taken from the arm of Edward Turner.—See cafe 22d.

FORTY-THIRD CASE.

Samuel Fairbrother began to be indifpofed on the 9th day, and had repeatedly flight feverifh paroxyfms, with pain in the axilla, till the 14th day, when four fmall puftules appeared, after which no farther complaint enfued.

FORTY FOURTH CASE.

In Richard Calloway the inoculated part tumified in the ufual manner, and on the 9th

day he firſt complained of a pain in the axilla
and head-ach, which continued till the 12th
day: an extenſive bright red bluſh then ſurrounded the tumour, and no farther complaint enſued. At this time alſo ſome puſtules appeared, but their number never exceeded twenty. He had been inoculated in
the hand as well as in the arm, in order to
diſcover if the appearance of the tumour in
a part conſtantly expoſed to the air would
be the ſame as in the arm kept covered by
his dreſs. The difference was very evident,
for the tumour upon his hand was much more
extenſive, of a more livid colour, and attended
with more inflammation than the other.

FORTY-FIFTH CASE.

James Camplin ſuffered rather more from the
eruptive complaints than Calloway, and they
continued with him a day longer. However
the

the difeafe gave him very little uneafinefs, and he had only thirty puftules.

———————

FORTY-SIXTH CASE.

John Turner's arm was inflamed very exten-fively, and he became feverifh on the 8th day. The following day many puftules appeared; and on the 11th day he was almoft covered with puftules, having about 1000. Thefe, however, were perfectly diftinct, and they all maturated favourably, fo that about the 17th day he was completely well.

———————

FORTY-SEVENTH & FORTY-EIGHTH CASE.

Joanna Buckley and Mary Welch had the difeafe in its mildeft form. On the 8th day an efflorefcence furrounded the inoculated part in both thefe children, and during this day only they appeared a little indifpofed. No puftules appeared upon either of them.

I 2   All

All the fix patients, thus infected with vaccine difeafe from E. Turner, were fubfequently inoculated with variolous matter, which did not produce any diforder.

———

February 18th, William Walker, eleven months old; February 24th, Sarah Dixon, nineteen years old; Thomas Elliftone, aged fifteen months; Maria Dunn, aged twenty months; and James Cummins, aged fourteen weeks, were all inoculated with the matter of Cow-pox taken from the arm of Hannah Bumpus.

———

FORTY-NINTH CASE.

* William Walker's arm tumified in the ufual

---

* The father of this child is an ingenious engraver in Rofamond Street, Clerkenwell, who having loft a child under the effects of the inoculated Small-pox, was induced to inoculate his only fon for the Cow-pox. The particulars of the cafe are related by Mr. Walker himfelf, in the Medical and Phyfical Journal for March 1799.

manner,

manner, but he did not manifeſt the leaſt
indiſpoſition during the courſe of the infection; neither did any puſtules appear, except
one or two at the inoculated part.

FIFTIETH CASE.

Sarah Dixon's arm tumified in the uſual
manner, and on the 10th day ſhe began to
complain of a pain in her head and loins;
this was followed by ſhiverings, and a pain
in the axilla, and acroſs her ſhoulders. 13th
day. The pains were much abated, and
ſome puſtules appeared. 16th day. She makes
no complaint, but of a ſoreneſs of her throat:
the eruption is now completed, and the number of the puſtules is found to be 174; all of
theſe afterwards maturated.

FIFTY-

FIFTY-FIRST CASE.

Thomas Elliftone was feverifh from the 6th to the 8th day, when the tumour was furrounded with an extenfive efflorefcence. After this time he had no ailment. No puftules appeared.

———

FIFTY-SECOND CASE.

Maria Dunn was hot and reftlefs from the fixth till the ninth day. She had no eruption.

———

FIFTY-THIRD CASE.

James Cummins did not feem the leaft difordered from the inoculation, although the inoculated part tumified very confiderably, and feveral puftules appeared at the margin of the tumour on the 11th day.

All the above mentioned perfons, inoculated with the matter of Cow-pox, taken from the

arm

arm of Bumpus, have been fince inoculated with variolous matter, but without effect.

———

John Giles, twenty years of age; **Wm.** Bigg, eighteen years old; William Briaris, fixteen years old; Sophia Dobinfon, five years old; Sarah Dobinfon, three years old; and Hannah Dobinfon, one year old, were inoculated with the matter of Cow-pox, taken from the arm of Jane Weft, February 21ft.

———

FIFTY-FOURTH CASE.

John Giles complained of head-ach from the 9th till the 11th day. A flight forenefs of the throat came on, and continued feveral days. He had about thirty puftules.

FIFTY-

FIFTY-FIFTH CASE.

William Bigg alſo complained of head-ach
and ſore throat ſeveral days, and had about
twelve puſtules.

———

FIFTY-SIXTH CASE.

Wm. Briaris firſt complained of indiſpoſition
on the 7th, and continued ſomewhat diſordered
till the 11th day. Only two puſtules appeared.

———

FIFTY-SEVENTH CASE.

Sophia Dobinſon's arm tumified extenſively,
but ſhe made no complaint during the whole
progreſs of the infection, and had no eruption.

———

FIFTY-EIGHTH CASE.

Sarah Dobinſon's caſe was in every reſpect
ſimilar to that of her ſiſter Sophia.

———

FIFTY-NINTH CASE.

Hannah Dobinſon ſuffered as little from the
diſeaſe

difeafe as either of her fifters, till the 14th day, when, according to her mother's report, fhe was feized with convulfive fits for two or three hours. She had no eruption.

The above fix patients have fince been inoculated for the Small-pox without effect.

———

Mary Grenville, twenty years old; Edward Honeywood, two years old; Thomas Rood, one year and a half old; Charlotte Mile, fifteen months old; John Jenkins, one year old; Henry Barber, eleven months old; Thomas Dix, eleven months old; Ann Walker, ten months old; Samuel Francis Brough, ten months old; Alexander Towfer, eight months old; Wm. Knighton, eight months old; Sarah Price, eight months old; Elizabeth Spilfbury, four months old; Elizabeth May, four months old; Mary Ann Sully, three months old; Francis Terry, two months old; Wm. Scott,

two

two months old; Wm. Johnſtone, two months old; and Mary Stewart, two months old, were inoculated with the matter of Cow-pox, taken from the arm of Martha Streeton, on February 25th.

SIXTIETH CASE.

Mary Grenville, on the 9th day, began to complain of head-ach, which continued till the 12th day, when a ſore throat came on, and gave her a little uneaſineſs for about two days. She had 35 puſtules.

SIXTY-FIRST CASE.

Edward Honeywood was not perceptibly diſordered from the inoculation, although his arm was much tumified; and on the 11th day it exhibited an effloreſcence. No eruption appeared.

SIXTY-SECOND CASE.

Thomas Rood was feveriſh from the 7th
till

till the 10th day, and at the commencement of the fever he had two or three short convulsive paroxysms; but no eruption took place.

SIXTY-THIRD CASE.

Charlotte Mile. A little redness was observed at the inoculated part on this child's arm for two or three days; but this had wholly disappeared on the seventh day, when she was inoculated with variolous matter, which produced the disease in a favourable manner.

SIXTY-FOURTH CASE.

John Jenkins became indisposed on the 12th day, and was very restless for three days. He had about 300 pustules.

SIXTY-FIFTH CASE.

Henry Barber had a slight fever on the eighth

day,

day, when fymptoms of dentition fupervened;
but the fever was of fhort duration. He had
but one puftule, and that was upon his
upper lip.

SIXTY-SIXTH CASE.

Thomas Dix's arm exhibited an extenfive
efflorefcence on the 11th day, and fome evanefcent puftules appeared; but he never mani-
fefted any indifpofition during the progrefs of
the infection.

SIXTY-SEVENTH CASE.

Ann Walker became indifpofed on the 9th
day, and continued fretful about 24 or 30
hours: the fever then ceafed, and fhe has
fince been wholly free from diforder. No
eruption appeared.

SIXTY-EIGHTH CASE.

Samuel Francis Brough was taken ill on the
9th day with fpafmodic paroxyfms, fucceeded

by

by fever: the former were of fhort duration, but the latter, with occafional intermiffions, continued for three days. 11th day. Some puftules appeared: their number, however, when the eruption was completed, did not exceed twenty.

SIXTY-NINTH CASE.

Alexander Towfer was reftlefs and feverifh about two days. Ten puftules appeared.

SEVENTIETH CASE.

William Knighton had no eruption. He was a little indifpofed between the feventh and tenth days.

SEVENTY-FIRST CASE.

Sarah Price had fome indifpofition on the 9th day, which terminated in a diarrhœa. On the 13th day fhe was perfectly well: two puftules were now difcovered upon her right foot, which were all fhe had.

SEVENTY-

SEVENTY-SECOND CASE.

Elizabeth Spilsbury was somewhat indisposed on the tenth, and on the fifteenth day; but the latter indisposition was the effect of teething. She had no eruption.

SEVENTY-THIRD CASE.

Elizabeth May was a little feverish on the eighth day, and continued somewhat restless till the 13th day: five pustules appeared.

SEVENTY-FOURTH CASE.

Mary Ann Sully was feverish on the 9th day, and passed a restless night, but on the next morning she was better: she made no farther complaint, and no pustules appeared.

SEVENTY-FIFTH CASE.

Francis Terry became feverish on the 9th day: the next morning a rash appeared, when he seemed to be as well as usual. He had only one pustule.

SEVENTY-

SEVENTY-SIXTH CASE.

William Scott was a little feverifh on the eighth day only : no eruption enfued.

SEVENTY-SEVENTH CASE.

William Johnfton's arm tumified in the ufual manner. He had no puftules, nor did he appear feverifh during the courfe of the difeafe ; but on the evening of the 13th day, he was thought to be a little reftlefs.

SEVENTY-EIGHTH CASE.

Mary Stewart, like Johnfton, was not perceptibly indifpofed during the whole progrefs of the infection, neither had fhe any puftules.

The above patients inoculated with the matter taken from Streeton, were fubfequently inoculated for the Small-pox, without affecting any but Charlotte Mile, in whom the inoculation for the Cow-pox took no effect.

February

February 27th, Joſeph Wrench, twenty-
four years old; Stephen Peters, nineteen
years old; Peter Peters, eighteen years old;
Elizabeth Brown, five years old; Mary
Shipley, three years old; Margaret Croſby,
ten months old; and John Evans, ſeven
months old, were inoculated with the matter
of Cow-pox, taken from the arm of James
Smith.

SEVENTY-NINTH CASE.

Joſeph Wrench continued indiſpoſed from
the 10th till the 13th day. An effloreſcence
appeared at the inoculated part on the 11th
day. 15th day. Several puſtules appeared,
and he now complained of a ſore throat,
which continued three days. The number of
the puſtules was thirty.

EIGHTIETH CASE.

Stephen Peters began to complain on the
eighth

eighth day, and continued to be affected with the ufual febrile fymptoms till the 13th day. He had only one puftule.

EIGHTY-FIRST CASE.

Peter Peter's complaints were fimilar to thofe in the preceding cafe. The efflorefcence did not appear till the 11th day. He had 24 puftules, all of which were very fmall.

EIGHTY-SECOND CASE.

Elizabeth Brown's tumour on the eighth day was furrounded by an efflorefcence. She made no complaint, nor had fhe any eruption.

EIGHTY-THIRD CASE.

Mary Shipley's arm exhibited an effloref-cence on the eighth day; but fhe was not perceptibly indifpofed, and had only one puftule.

L   EIGHTY-

EIGHTY-FOURTH CASE.

Margaret Crofby had no eruption, nor was she perceptibly ill during the progrefs of her inoculation. Her arm, however, tumified in the ufual manner, and difplayed an efflorefcence.

EIGHTY-FIFTH CASE.

On John Evan's arm there was an efflorefcence on the 6th day, and the following day a flight fever commenced with a fpafmodic paroxyfm, but he was perfectly well on the ninth, and no eruption took place.

The above five perfons have been fince inoculated with variolous matter without effect.

Sarah Hat, twenty years old, and Elizabeth Platford, feventeen years old, were inoculated with matter of the Cow-pox, taken from the arm of Maria Murrell.

EIGHTY-

EIGHTY-SIXTH CASE.

Sarah Hat began to complain on the 6th day, and fhe continued much indifpofed till the 11th day, when the tumour was furrounded by an efflorefcence, and fhe made no farther complaint. The number of the puftules which appeared was about forty.

EIGHTY-SEVENTH CASE.

Elizabeth Platford was taken ill on the 9th day, when fhe complained of pain in the head and loins, with chillinefs, &c. : the inoculated part at this time was confiderably inflamed : the tumour was circular, but flat, and not fur-rounded by any efflorefcence. 11th day. The pains and fhiverings continue: pulfe very frequent and weak: tongue white. 13th day. The fymptoms ftill continue: fhe alfo complains of pain acrofs her fhoulders: fome puftules appear. 15th day. She complains of pain in the loins, and of giddinefs: the number of the puftules

is

is much increafed. 17th day. The pains continue: fhe is very weak and faint: her eyes and throat are inflamed and painful: the edges of the tumour are befet with confluent puftules: the puftules upon her face are about 2 or 300, and approach to confluency. 19th day. Her face is confiderably fwelled, and the puftules are now maturating rapidly. She makes no complaint, but of the forenefs occafioned by the eruption. 21ft day. Swelling of the face much fubfided: the puftules in a ftate of deficcation. 23d day. She continues recovering. 26th day. She complains of a fore throat, and a cough is troublefome to her. 28th day. The fore throat is almoft gone, but the cough continues: pulfe 100. 30th day. The cough is ftill violent. 32d day. The cough is abated, and her appetite improves: from this time fhe gradually recovered.

Both the above patients were afterwards inoculated

culated with variolous matter which produced no effect.

Isaac Cowling, twenty-three years old; Mary Webb, twelve years old; Sophia Mason, two years and a half old; and Elizabeth Goodluck, three months old, were, on the 2d of March, inoculated for the Cow-pox, with matter taken from the arm of G. Reed.

EIGHTY-EIGHTH CASE.

Isaac Cowling sickened on the 9th, and the eruptive complaints did not wholly go off till the 14th day. He had about 50 pustules.

EIGHTY-NINTH CASE.

Mary Webb began to complain on the 7th day, and continued feverish for a week. On the 10th day a redness was diffused over the greatest part of her arm, between the elbow and shoulder, and did not wholly disappear till the 14th day. She had about 12 pustules.

NINTIETH

NINETIETH CASE.

Sophia Mafon's arm tumified in the ufual way, and exhibited an efflorefcence on the 10th day. She had four or five fmall evanefcent puftules, but did not feem indifpofed during the courfe of the infeƐion.

NINETY-FIRST CASE.

Elizabeth Goodluck was taken ill on the 8th day, when fhe had a flight fpafmodic fit: the tumour at this time exhibited an efflorefcence. 11th day. Has had no indifpofition fince yefterday. No eruption took place.

None of the above three patients took the Small-pox in confequence of inoculation with variolous matter.

NINETY-SECOND and NINETY-THIRD CASE.

March 3d.—C. S. Cooke, four years old; and A. T. Cooke, two years old, were inoculated with the matter of Cow-pox, taken from the arm of George Meacock.

An

An efflorefcence at the inoculated part took place in both thefe children on the 10th day, but neither of them feemed indifpofed from the inoculation, nor did any puftules appear upon them. They were alfo put to the teft of inoculation with variolous matter, but no difeafe enfued.

———

March 3d,—A. K. Gunter, one year old; Matthew Sears, nine months old; and Eliz. Giles, nine months old, were inoculated with the matter of Cow-pox, taken from the arm of H. Dobinfon.

———

NINETY-FOURTH CASE.

A. K. Gunter was a little feverifh for two days. On the 10th day the tumour was furrounded by an efflorefcence, which became very extenfive. Only two or three imperfect puftules appeared.

NINETY-

NINETY-FIFTH CASE.

Matthew Sears was indifpofed for about four or five days. The tumour was fmall and angular, nor was it ever furrounded with an efflorefcence. He had about 200 puftules.

NINETY-SIXTH CASE.

Elizabeth Giles became indifpofed on the 10th day. The tumour had a dark red coloured border without any efflorefcence. She had from 70 to 100 puftules.

The above patients have been inoculated with variolous matter without effect.

Richard Scott, two years and a half old; Sarah Bennett, one year old; Maria Black, one year old; Mary Jenkins, nine months old; John Lawyer, eight months old; Eliz. King, fix months old; William Jones, fix months old; Efther Phipps, fix months old;

Thomas

Thomas Newman, fix months old; and Ann Harper, five months old, were inoculated with the matter of Cow-pox, taken from the arm of Elizabeth Brown.

NINETY-SEVENTH CASE.

Richard Scott became feverifh for a fhort time on the tenth day. He had about 14 puftules.

NINETY-EIGHTH CASE.

Elizabeth King's tumour, on the 9th day, was furrounded with an efflorefcence. She did not manifeft any indifpofition, nor had any eruption.

99th,—100th,—and 101ft CASES.

The cafes of John Lawyer, William Jones, and Sarah Bennett, were fimilar to that of King.

M   ONE

ONE HUNDRED and SECOND CASE.

Eſther Phipps was a little reſtleſs and feveriſh from the 10th till the 13th day, but had no eruption.

———

ONE HUNDRED and THIRD CASE.

Maria Black became feveriſh on the ninth day, and was indiſpoſed for two or three days, during which time ſhe had two ſlight convulſions. Some puſtules appeared, but did not ſuppurate.

———

ONE HUNDRED and FOURTH CASE.

Mary Jenkins was a little indiſpoſed on the tenth day. She had no eruption.

———

ONE HUNDRED and FIFTH CASE.

Ann Harper was a little reſtleſs during the ſeventh and eighth night; but no eruption took place.

ONE

ONE HUNDRED and SIXTH CASE.

Thomas Newman was feverifh from the feventh till the twelfth day; but no puftules appeared.

———

March 4th, George Paul, three years old, Ann Paul, one year old; Martha Chandler, five months old; Martha Hat, one year old; Eliza. Boardore, feven months old; Samuel Lampart, two years old; Ann Page, one year and a half old; Jane Carter, five weeks old; William New, eighteen months old; Sufan Sermon, fix months old; Alice Marfhall, two years old; Harriot Marfhall, four months old; and Frances Henley, five years old, were inoculated with the matter of Cow-pox, taken from the arm of Elizabeth May.

———

ONE HUNDRED and SEVENTH CASE.

George Paul was not perceptibly indifpofed from the inoculation. He had two puftules.

ONE HUNDRED and EIGHTH CASE.

Ann Paul was feverifh for about three days, and had forty puftules, all of which were much fmaller than thofe of the Small-pox.

ONE HUNDRED and NINTH CASE.

Martha Chandler's inoculation produced a very extenfive efflorefcence; but neither fever nor eruption enfued.

ONE HUNDRED and TENTH CASE.

Martha Hat did not become indifpofed till the thirteenth day, when a few fmall puftules appeared.

ONE HUNDRED and ELEVENTH CASE.

Elizabeth Boardore's arm tumified confider-ably; but neither efflorefcence, fever, nor eruption, took place.

ONE

ONE HUNDRED and TWELFTH CASE.

Samuel Lampart was fomewhat difordered from the 9th till the 12th day, and had three fmall imperfect puftules.

———

ONE HUNDRED and THIRTEENTH CASE.

Ann Page was not fenfibly indifpofed from the inoculation, neither had fhe any eruption. The tumour was furrounded with an effloref-cence on the 12th day.

———

ONE HUNDRED and FOURTEENTH CASE.

Jane Carter was flightly indifpofed from the 7th till the 10th day, and had two or three puftules.

———

ONE HUNDRED and FIFTEENTH CASE.

William New was ill four days, and had about 100 puftules.

ONE

ONE HUNDRED and SIXTEENTH CASE.

Susan Sermon was taken ill on the 9th day,
when she vomited. She continued feverish till
the 12th day. Only five pustules appeared.

––––––

117th,—118th,—and 119th CASES.

Alice Marshall, Frances Henley, and Harriet
Marshall had no eruption, nor appeared to
have any disorder from the inoculation. The
local disease, however, was considerable in
all these patients, and was attended with an
efflorescence.

All the above patients who received the
infection from Brown and May, have since
been inoculated for the Small-pox without
effect.

––––––

ONE HUNDRED and TWENTIETH CASE.

Mary Crouch, aged three years, was inoculated with matter taken from one of the
pustules

pustules upon John Turner, (fee Cafe 46th). A tumour formed at the inoculated part in the usual manner, which was furrounded with an efflorefcence; but neither fever nor erruption took place.

121ft and 122d CASES.

Elizabeth Wood, aged three years, and Wm. Clifford, two years and a half old, were inoculated with Cow-pox matter, taken from the arm of Mary Stewart, March 4th. Both thefe children were flightly indifpofed about the 10th day, but neither of them had any pustules.

March 6th. The following perfons were inoculated with the matter of Cow-pox, taken from the arm of Ann Walker.

Amelia Reftieux, four months old; John Bates, fix weeks old; Martha Thompfon,

two

two years old; William London, three years
old; James London, fix months old; Frances
Wallace, three years old; Jofeph Rogers,
forty-two years old; Thomas Thoroughgood,
fourteen years old; and Ann Thoroughgood,
feventeen years old.

———

123d and 124th CASES.

Amelia Reſtieux and John Bates, neither
experienced any diforder from the inoculation, nor had any eruption; but both their
arms tumified in the ufual manner.

———

ONE HUNDRED & TWENTY-FIFTH CASE.

Martha Thompfon was feverifh from the
8th till the 10th day. She had only one
puſtule.

———

ONE HUNDRED & TWENTY-SIXTH CASE.

William London was taken ill on the 10th
day, and vomited, but the following day was
as well as ufual. He had no eruption.

ONE

ONE HUNDRED & TWENTY-SEVENTH CASE.
James London had no perceptible diforder;
and no puftules appeared. On the 10th day
the tumour was furrounded with an efflorefcence.

ONE HUNDRED & TWENTY-EIGHTH CASE.
Frances Wallace was feverifh for two or
three days, but no eruption enfued.

ONE HUNDRED & TWENTY-NINTH CASE.
Jofeph Rogers on the 8th day complained
of pain in the axilla, and was affected with
head-ach for two or three days; but he had
no eruption.

ONE HUNDRED & THIRTIETH CASE.
Thomas Thoroughgood made the fame
complaints as Rogers. He had 33 puftules.

ONE HUNDRED & THIRTY-FIRST CASE.
Ann Thoroughgood was indifpofed for fix
or feven days, but fhe had only ten puftules.

The preceding twelve patients have had variolous matter inferted in their arms without effect.

————

The following perfons were inoculated with the matter taken from the puftules of Martha Streeton, viz.

Sufan Reeve, eighteen months old; Ann Reeve, five weeks old; Sufan Richardfon, thirteen years old; and Mary Adams, fix months old.

————

132d and 133d CASES.

Sufan Reeve and Ann Reeve were very little difordered by the inoculation; the former, however, had 20, and the latter 12 puftules.

————

ONE HUNDRED & THIRTY-FOURTH CASE.

Sufan Richardfon continued indifpofed from the 10th till the 14th day, but fhe had only 12 puftules.

ONE

ONE HUNDRED & THIRTY-FIFTH CASE.

Mary Adams had about 200 puftules; but the eruptive fymptoms were not fevere. The tumour in this cafe fpread, and formed an irregular margin, which was ftudded with confluent puftules.

———

March 7th.—The difeafe was transferred from the puftules upon Sarah Dixon, to the following children, viz.

Caroline Harrifkind, four years old; Wm. Harrifkind, two years old; Daniel Harding, fourteen weeks old; Elizabeth Harding, three years old; James Waters, twelve years old; and Jofeph Harding, feventeen years old.

———

136th and 137th CASES.

Caroline and Wm. Harrifkind were feverifh for two or three days. The former had 100, and the latter had 12 puftules.

138th

138th and 139th CASES.

Daniel and Elizabeth Harding were but
very flightly indifpofed from the inoculation.
Daniel had 15 very fmall puftules; Elizabeth
had only two.

ONE HUNDRED & FORTIETH CASE.

James Waters complained of head-ach,
pains of his limbs, and fore throat, from the
8th till the 14th day. The tumour at the
inoculated part was never much elevated
above the fkin, and had an angulated border.
He had 120 puftules.

ONE HUNDRED & FORTY-FIRST CASE.

Jofeph Harding was very flightly difordered, and had no puftules.

March 8th.—William Shipton, four years
old; George Staits, two years old; Elizabeth
Youngman, three months old; Mary Dudley,

two

two years old; William Cade, ten months old; and William Piper, four months old, were inoculated with the matter of Cow-pox, taken from the arm of Efther Phipps.

142d,—143d,—144th,—and 145th CASES.

William Shipton, Elizabeth Youngman, William Cade, and William Piper, had no puftules; and none of them appeared to be difordered from the inoculation, except Piper, who was a little feverifh on the 8th day. An efflorefcence took place around the tumour in all of them.

ONE HUNDRED & FORTY-SIXTH CASE.

George Staits was indifpofed for two days, and had 3 or 4 fmall puftular eruptions.

ONE HUNDRED & FORTY-SEVENTH CASE.

Mary Dudley was a little feverifh on the 9th day, when a rafh appeared which receded

the

the following day, and about 50 fmall puftules were difcovered; thefe, however, difappeared in the courfe of 24 hours.

———

March 11th.—Hannah Timms, nineteen years old; Sufan Timms, feventeen years old; Jane Franklin, twelve years old; and Henry Lee, fifteen years old, were inoculated with the matter of Cow-pox, taken from the arm of Mary Webb.

———

ONE HUNDRED & FORTY-EIGHTH CASE.

Hannah Timms was affected with febrile fymptoms from the 8th till the 16th day, and had 165 puftules, all of which fuppurated.

———

ONE HUNDRED & FORTY-NINTH CASE.

Sufan Timms was ill from the 9th till the 14th day. She had no eruption.

Jane

ONE HUNDRED & FIFTIETH CASE.

Jane Franklin was very little indifpofed from the inoculation, and had no eruption.

ONE HUNDRED & FIFTY-FIRST CASE.

Henry Lee complained for two or three days, and had only one puftule.

March 13th.—The following perfons were inoculated with the matter of Cow-pox, taken from the arm of Sarah Hat, viz.

Ann Spooner, twenty-one years old; Matthew Wall, fourteen years old; John Wall, ten years old; William Ockendon, twelve years old; Jofeph Ockendon, ten years old; William Jennings, feven years old; George Jennings, fix years old; John Pluckrofe, feven years old; Charlotte Webb, fourteen weeks old; Charles Dibden, three months old; Elizabeth Eaton, two years old;

Charlotte

Charlotte Eaton, ten months old ; and Joſeph Pigg, eleven years old.

ONE HUNDRED & FIFTY-SECOND CASE.

Ann Spooner was indiſpoſed for three or four days, and had 150 puſtules.

ONE HUNDRED & FIFTY-THIRD CASE.

Matthew Wall was a little indiſpoſed for three days. He had 10 puſtules.

ONE HUNDRED & FIFTY-FOURTH CASE.

John Wall made no complaint, and had no eruption.

ONE HUNDRED & FIFTY-FIFTH CASE.

William Ockendon was indiſpoſed from the 8th till the 10th day. He had only one puſtule.

ONE

ONE HUNDRED & FIFTY-SIXTH CASE.

Jóſeph Ockendon was ill for three days.
He had no eruption.

ONE HUNDRED & FIFTY-SEVENTH CASE.

William Jennings complained of head-ach
two days. He had only one puſtule.

ONE HUNDRED & FIFTY-EIGHTH CASE.

George Jennings was diſordered in the ſame
manner as his brother William, but he had no
eruption.

ONE HUNDRED & FIFTY-NINTH CASE.

John Pluckroſe made no complaint, and had
no eruption.

160th and 161ſt CASES.

Charlotte Webb and Charles Dibden.—The
former was not perceptibly diſordered by the
inoculation, and had no puſtules. The latter
was a little feveriſh on the ninth day, and
o   vomited.

vomited. He had three puſtules at the inoculated part only.

162d and 163d CASES.

Elizabeth Eaton and Charles Eaton were
both ſlightly indiſpoſed on the 11th and 12th
day; and each had about twenty puſtules.

ONE HUNDRED & SIXTY-FOURTH CASE.

Joſeph Pigg complained of a pain in the
axilla, and of a ſlight head-ach for four days.
He had fourteen puſtules only.

March 13th.—The following were inoculated with the matter of Cow-pox, taken from
the arm of Samuel Lampart, viz.

Mary Ockendon, ſixteen years old; Sarah
Ockendon, ſeven years old; Sarah Stacey,
twelve years old; Ann Stacey, ſeven years
old; Mary Fuller, eleven years old; Iſabella
Barrett, eleven years old; Mary Perry, three
years

years old; Suſaн Vinicum, five months old; Elizabeth Renſden, eighteen months old; Mary Ward, ten months old; Wm. Terrey, two months old; Caroline Poorey, three years old; Ann Poorey, eleven months old; John Langſtaff, four years and an half old; Emma Lightfoot, thirteen months old; Daniel Sinclair, ſeven months old; M. H. Hills, eighteen weeks old; and Catharine Donaldſon, nineteen months old.

ONE HUNDRED & SIXTY FIFTH CASE.
Mary Ockendon was indiſpoſed from the 9th till the 14th day. She had only ſix puſtules.

ONE HUNDRED & SIXTY-SIXTH CASE.
Sarah Ockendon complained of head-ach, pain of her limbs, &c. from the 10th till the 14th day, but only four puſtules appeared.

ONE HUNDRED & SIXTY-SEVENTH CASE.
Sarah Stacey was indiſpoſed from the 10th till the 15th day. No puſtules appeared.

ONE

ONE HUNDRED & SIXTY-EIGHTH CASE.

Ann Stacey's cafe was fimilar to that of her fifter Sarah.

169th and 170th CASES.

Mary Fuller and Ifabella Barrett, both complained of the febrile fymptoms from the 9th till the 14th day. The former had fix, and the latter twenty puftules.

171ft,—172d,—and 173d CASES.

Mary Perry, Sufan Vinicum, and Elizabeth Brenfden, did not appear to be indifpofed from the inoculation, and had no eruption: but the tumours in all were confiderable, and furrounded by an efflorefcence.

ONE HUNDRED & SEVENTY-FOURTH CASE.

Mary Ward was a little feverifh for two days, and a few fmall puftules appeared for one day only.

175th,

175th,—176th,—177th, and 178th CASES.

Wm. Terry, Ann Poorey, Caroline Poorey, and John Langftaff, had no puftules, neither did any of them appear to be indifpofed, except Ann Poorey, who was feverifh for two days.

———

179th and 180th CASES.

Emma Lightfoot and Daniel Sinclair were both a little difordered for two or three days, and the former had four or five fmall puftules, but the latter had no eruption.

———

181ft and 182d CASES.

Ann Hills and Catharine Donaldfon had neither fever nor eruption.

———

ONE HUNDRED & EIGHTY-THIRD CASE.

Ann Clarke was inoculated with the matter of Cow-pox, taken from the arm of Peter Peters, which produced two or three fmall evanefcent puftules; but no fever took place.

March

March 15th.—John Buckthorpe, twenty-two years old; John Cater, fourteen years of age; Sufan Tomlins, nineteen years old; Maria Burgefs, four years old; and Sophia Burgefs, three years old, were inoculated for the Cow-pox, with matter taken from the arm of Jofeph Wrench.

ONE HUNDRED & EIGHTY-FOURTH CASE.

John Buckthorpe was indifpofed from the 9th till the 14th day. He had nearly 100 puftules.

ONE HUNDRED & EIGHTY FIFTH CASE.

John Cater complained of head-ach, &c. from the 8th till the 11th day. He had forty puftules.

ONE HUNDRED & EIGHTY-SIXTH CASE.

Sufan Tomlins continued ill for three days. She had 24 puftules.

187th

187th and 188th CASES.

Maria and Sophia Burgefs were neither indifpofed from the inoculation. Sophia had
no puftules, and Maria only three.

March 18.—The following perfons were
inoculated with the matter of Cow-pox, taken
from the arm of Elizabeth Platford.

John Williams, feven months old; James
Runtfman, three months old; Robert Lear,
feventeen months old; John Selby, five
months old; Samuel Ariell, two years old;
James Ariell, five years old; Henry Servy,
two years and a half old; Sarah Lovell, four
years old; Henry Lovell, two years old;
Rebecca Salmon, nine months old; John
Corwell, eight months old; and Francis Cundell, fix months old.

ONE

ONE HUNDRED & EIGHTY-NINTH CASE.

John Williams had no indifpofition, nor no puftules. The tumour was furrounded with an efflorefcence on the 11th day.

ONE HUNDRED & NINETIETH CASE.

James Runtfman was a little feverifh on the evening of the 10th. He had no eruption.

ONE HUNDRED & NINETY FIRST CASE.

Robert Lear's cafe was fimilar to that of Runtfman.

ONE HUNDRED & NINETY-SECOND CASE.

John Selby was feverifh two days, and had forty puftules.

193d and 194th CASES.

Samuel Ariell and James Ariell were both feverifh on the 10th and 11th day, but neither had any eruption.

ONE

195th and 196th CASES.

Henry Servy and Sarah Lovell were difordered two days. The former had no puftules, the latter 40.

ONE HUNDRED & NINETY-SEVENTH CASE.

Henry Lovell was ill three days, and had 170 puftules.

ONE HUNDRED & NINETY-EIGHTH CASE.

Rebecca Salmon was very flightly indifpofed, but had about 200 puftules, which were very fmall.

199th and 200th CASES.

John Corwell and Francis Cundell were both feverifh for two or three days: the former had 36, and the latter 12 puftules.

All the above patients, inoculated fince the 6th of March, have fubfequently had variolous matter inferted in their arms, except the two Ariells, but it produced no diforder.

P   In

In order that the progreſſive deſcent of the
Cow-pox infection from patient to patient,
as well as the magnitude of the diſeaſe which
was excited by the inoculation, may be comprehended at one view, I have ſubjoined the
following tabular ſtatement.

It may be obſerved, that the matter uſed
for the preceding inoculations, was not only
derived immediately from the puſtular eruptions upon the teats of the cow, but alſo from
Sarah Rice, who contracted the diſeaſe by
milking the infected cows. I begin with the
former. In the firſt and ſecond diviſions op-
poſite to the names, the age in years or
months is recorded; in the third, the number of days during which the febrile ſymptoms
continued; and in the laſt, the number of
puſtules produced.

TABLE.

T A B L E.

From the Cow to	Years of Age	Months	Days of Illnefs.	No. of puftules
M. Payne . .	2	6	3	0
E. Payne . .	—	4	5	0
Buckland . .	—	4	+	24
R. Payne . .	10	—	0	5
Redding . .	16	—	1	4
Collingridge . .	17	—	4	170
Pink . . .	15	—	0	0
From M. and E. PAYNE to				
Talley . . .	14	—	—	—
Brown . .	15	—	—	—
From COLLINGRIDGE to				
Mundy . . .	25	—	2	15
George . . .	25	—	6	530
Butcher . .	13	—	2	0
Dorfet . . .	19	—	1	0
From BUCKLAND's puftules to				
S. Price . .	13	—	2	6
From REDDING to				
Wife . .	14	—	0	4
From MUNDY to				
Slade . . .	21	—	5	4
From GEORGE to				
Tarrent . . .	19	—	1	0

	Age Years.	Months	Days of Illnefs.	No. of Puftules.
From BUTCHER to				
Jewel	20	—	2	0
Bumpus	20	—	6	310
Weft	21	—	5	20
W. Hull	11	—	4	200
H. Hull	13	—	1	8
S. Hull	8	—	2	120
From JEWEL to				
Fifk	—	4	4	40
Reed	15	—	5	70
From S. PRICE to				
Pedder	—	11	5	40
Hoole	—	5	5	102
Hickland	—	6	3	300
Morton	—	9	7	200
From FISK to				
Davy	—	3	1	3
Murrell	—	7	4	20
From BUMPUS to				
Dixon	19	—	4	174
W. Walker	—	11	0	0
Cummins	—	3	0	0
Elliftone	—	3	2	0
Dunn	—	8	3	0
From WEST to				
So. Dobinfon	5	—	0	0
Sarah Dobinfon	3	—	0	0
H. Dobinfon	1	—	1	0
Giles	20	—	3	30

	Age, Years.	Months.	Days of Illness.	No. of Pustules.
From WEST to				
Bigg . .	18	—	5	12
Briaris . .	16	—	4	2
From REED to				
Cowling . . .	23	—	4	50
Webb . . .	12	—	0	12
Maſon . . .	2	6	0	4
Goodluck . .	—	3	2	0
From MURRELL to				
Hatt . . .	20	—	4	40
Platford . . .	17	—	8	1000
From H. DOBINSON to				
Gunter . . .	1	—	2	3
Sears . . .	—	9	5	200
E. Giles . . .	—	9	3	90
From DIXON's Puſtules to				
C. Harriſkind . .	4	—	4	100
W. Harriſkind . .	2	~	3	12
D. Harding . .	—	3	1	15
E. Harding . .	3	—	1	2
Waters . .	12	—	6	120
J. Harding . .	17	—	1	0
From WEBB to .				
H. Timms . .	19	—	7	165
S. Timms . .	17	—	5	0
Franklin . . .	12	—	1	0
Lee . .	15	—	2	3
From HAT to				
Spooner . .	21	—	4	150

	Age, Years.	Months.	Days of Illness.	No. of Pustules.
From HAT to				
M. Wall	14	—	3	10
J. Wall	10	—	0	0
J. Ockendon	10	—	3	0
W. Ockendon	12	—	3	1
W. Jennings	7	—	2	1
G. Jennings	6	—	2	0
Pluckrofe	7	—	0	0
C. Webb	—	3	0	0
Dibden	—	3	1	0
E. Eaton	2	—	2	2
C. Eaton	—	10	2	2
Pigg	11	—	4	14
From PLATFORD to				
Williams	—	7	0	0
Runtfman	—	3	1	0
Lear	1	5	1	0
Selby	—	5	2	40
S. Ariell	2	—	2	0
J. Ariell	5	—	2	0
Servy	2	6	2	0
S. Lovell	4	—	2	40
H. Lovell	2	—	3	170
Salmon	—	9	1	200
Corwell	—	8	3	36
Cundell	—	6	2	12
From S. RICE to				
Harris	21	—	0	300
Bunker	15	—	3	3

	Age, Years.	Months.	Days of Illnefs.	No. of Puftules.
From S. Rice to				
Crouch	7	—	0	0
Fox	25	—	—	—
Dennis	23	—	—	—
From Crouch to				
Keys	25	—	1	0
Turner	24	—	6	220
Morgan	1	—	5	0
Mr. Coleman's Cow.				
From the Cow to				
Streeton	22	—	6	300
Smith	16	—	4	105
Meacock	30	—	5	350
From Turner to				
Fairbrother	15	—	4	4
Calloway	19	—	3	20
Camplin	17	—	4	30
J. Turner	—	8	2	1000
Buckley	—	5	1	0
Welch	—	3	1	0
From Streeton to				
Grenvill	20	—	5	35
Honeywood	2	—	0	0
Rood	1	6	2	0
Mile	1	3	0	0
Jenkins	1	—	3	300
Barber	—	11	2	1
Dix	—	11	0	6
A. Walker	—	10	2	0

	Age, Years.	Months.	Days of Illnefs.	No. of Puftules.
From STREETON to				
Brough . . .	—	10	3	20
Towfer . . .	—	8	2	10
Knighton . . .	—	8	2	0
Price . . .	—	8	1	0
Spilfbury . . .	—	4	2	0
May . .	—	4	4	5
Sully . .	—	3	1	0
Terry . . .	—	2	1	1
Scott . .	—	2	1	0
Johnfton . .	—	2	0	0
Stewart . . .	—	2	0	0
From SMITH to				
Wrench . . .	24	—	3	30
S. Peters . .	19	—	4	1
P. Peters . .	18	—	4	24
Brown . . .	5	—	0	0
Shipley . .	3	—	0	1
Crofby . .	—	10	0	0
Evans . .	—	7	2	0
From MEACOCK to				
C. Cooke . .	4	—	0	0
A. Cooke . .	2	—	0	0
From BROWN to				
R. Scott . . .	2	6	1	14
Bennett . . .	1	—	0	0
Black . . .	1	—	3	7
M. Jenkins . .	—	9	1	0
Lawyer . . .	—	8	0	0

	Age, Years.	Months.	Days of Illnefs.	No. of Puftules.
From BROWN to				
King	—	6	0	0
Jones	—	6	0	0
Phipps	—	6	3	0
Newman	—	6	4	0
Harper	—	5	2	0
From MAY to				
G. Paul	3	—	0	2
A. Paul	1	—	3	40
Chandler	—	5	0	0
M. Hatt	1	—	1	5
Boardore	—	7	0	0
Lampart	2	—	2	3
Page	1	6	0	0
Carter	—	1	2	3
Sermon	—	6	3	5
A. Marſhall	2	—	0	0
H. Marſhall	—	4	0	0
Henley	5	—	0	0
New	1	6	4	100
From TURNER's Puſtules to				
M. Crouch	3	—	0	0
From STEWART to				
Wood	3	—	1	0
Clifford	2	6	1	0
From A. WALKER to				
Reſtieux	—	4	0	0
Bates	—	$1\frac{1}{2}$	0	0
Thompſon	2	—	2	1

	Age, Years.	Months.	Days of Illness.	No. of Pustules.
From A. WALKER to				
W. London . .	3	—	1	0
J. London . .	—	6	0	0
Wallace . . .	3	—	2	0
Rogers . . .	42	—	3	0
T. Thoroughgood . .	14	—	3	33
A. Thoroughgood .	17	—	6	10
From STREETON's pustules to				
S. Reeve . . .	1	6	1	20
A. Reeve . .	—	1	1	12
Richardson . .	13	—	3	12
Adams . . .	—	6	3	200
From PHIPPS to				
Shipton . . .	4	—	0	0
Staits . . .	2	—	2	3
Youngman	—	3	0	0
Dudley . . .	2	—	1	50
Cade . . .	—	10	0	0
Piper . . .	—	4	1	0
From LAMPART to				
M. Ockendon . .	16	—	4	6
S. Ockendon . .	17	—	3	4
S. Stacey . . .	12	—	4	0
A. Stacey . . .	7	—	4	0
Fuller . . .	11	—	4	6
Barrett . . .	11	—	4	20
Perry . . .	3	—	0	0
Vinicum . .	—	5	0	0
Bensden . . .	1	6	0	0

	Age, Years.	Months.	Days of Illness.	No. of Pustules.
From LAMPART to				
Ward	—	10	2	7
Terry	—	2	0	0
C. Poorey	3	—	0	0
A. Poorey	—	11	2	0
Langſtaff	4	6	0	0
Lightfoot	1	1	2	5
Sinclair	—	7	2	0
Hills	—	4	0	0
Donaldſon	1	7	0	0
From WRENCH to				
Buckthorpe	22	—	4	100
Cater	14	—	3	40
Tomlin	19	—	3	24
M. Burgeſs	4	—	0	3
S. Burgeſs	3	—	0	0
From P. PETERS to				
Clarke	5	—	0	3

The preceding Table comprehends all the Caſes originally intended to have been given in this work, the publication of which from a concurrence of circumſtances, has been delayed much longer than the Author expected, and has thereby afforded him an opportunity of making the following additions.

Q 2

	Age, Years.	Months.	Days of Illnefs.	No. of Puftules.
From PLATFORD's puftules to				
Prince . . .	1	—	0	30
Chandler . . .	1	9	0	40
Jervoife . . .	—	6	1	0
Palmer . . .	—	3	3	100
Henderfon . .	—	10	4	300
Crawford . .	1	10	3	250
From DUDLEY to				
A. Vallentine . .	3	—	2	0
J. Vallentine . .	2	—	3	0
From S. TIMMS to				
S. Harris . . .	21	—	7	6
S. Clarke . . .	—	9	2	0
M. Harris . .	23	—	6	60
Ludgrove . .	—	11	2	0
Stringer . . .	20	—	4	2
From GRENVILLE to				
B. Crane . . .	2	—	3	200
T. Crane . . .	4	—	2	12
Garrett . . .	14	—	4	62
M. Crane . .	8	—	4	30
From A. STACEY to				
M. Stacey . .	38	—	3	5
R. Stacey . .	—	7	0	12
J. Stacey . . .	3	6	0	5
Harriott . . .	—	8	1	6
M. Waite . . .	—	10	2	50
J. Waite . . .	3	—	2	20

	Age, Years.	Months.	Days of Illness.	No. of Pustules.
From M. OCKENDON to				
H. Pigley	22	—	4	100
Dach	—	4½	2	0
G. Pigley	—	5	0	0
Morgan	—	2½	0	0
Bradley	19	—	6	156
Harrifon	—	2	1	0
Morton	—	5	0	0
Cooper	4	11	0	0
E. Cooper	—	4	1	0
Ellikins	3	3	0	0
M. Hide	4	11	0	0
D. Hide	1	5	0	0
Phillips	—	8	0	0
From TOMLIN to				
C. Hopes	3	—	1	0
S. Hopes	1	—	0	0
Oliphant	3	—	1	0
Caftin	—	6	3	0
Hamm	2	—	0	0
A. Smith	4	—	0	0
Reynolds	—	4	0	0
From J. WALL to				
Gallway	—	3	1	0
Barneby	1	6	0	0
Dick	2	8	0	3
Dalkins	—	5½	1	0
Bromley	1	2	2	3
Ford	—	6	2	0

	Age, Years.	Months.	Days of Illnefs.	No. of Puftules.
From J. VALLENTINE to				
Merrin . . .	—	3	0	0
Loathis . . .	4	—	3	5
Gedge . . .	—	4½	0	0
Beafley . . .	—	3	0	4
Goodman . . .	1	10	2	40
From SPOONER to				
Stainer . . .	16	—	3	34
. Pepler . .	4	—	0	0
Swannell . . .	10	—	3	6
F. Pepler . . .	2	—	0	0
Brown . . .	19	—	4	35
P. Roberts . .	6	—	4	12
M. Roberts . .	4	—	0	6
C. Roberts . .	1	8	3	6
Freeman . . .	11	—	4	40
A. Palmer . .	—	9	2	40
Wade . . .	16	—	4	3
From COOPER to				
Munden . . .	—	7	1	50
From H. TIMMS's puftules to				
Stiles . . .	—	6	3	500
Burrows . . .	—	5	1	12
From M. BARTLETT to				
J. Mundy . . .	—	6	3	100
From COWLEY to				
Nafh . . .	15	—	1	0
From SPOONER's puftules to				
Serjeant . . .	16	—	4	35

	Age, Years.	Months	Days of Illnefs.	No. of Puftules.
From SPOONER's Puftules to				
Cook . . .	15	—	2	11
From STRINGER's puftules to				
Argant . . .	17	—	7	19
From H. TIMMS's Puftules to				
E. Gilbert . .	17	—	3	4
Brewfter . . .	11	—	4	6
Truluck . . .	—	6	2	250
Wiggins . . .	—	5	0	7
Th. Turner . .	—	6	0	50
Gilbert . . .	—	6	3	500
Downes . . .	—	4	2	30
King . . .	—	2	2	4
Talbot . . .	—	4	3	500
From CORWELL to				
Graham . . .	—	4	0	0
Sellers . . .	15	—	0	0
From BARRETT to				
T. Barrett .	32	—	3	200
M. Barrett .	5	—	0	0
J. Barrett . . .	2	3	1	0
H. Barrett . .	—	7	2	30
E. Wybrow . .	5	—	3	200
T. Wybrow . .	9	—	3	150
J. Wybrow . .	1	—	1	6
Harwood . . .	2	3	1	6
M. Harwood . .	4	—	0	12
J. Harwood . .	5	—	2	6
P. Harwood : .	—	5	4	200

	Age, Years.	Months	Days of Illnefs.	No. of Puftules.
From BARRETT to				
Higgins . . .	—	3	0	0
M. Higgins . .	2	6	0	5
From HENDERSON to				
Upftone . . .	19	—	5	12
I. Bumpus . . .	16	—	5	20
From S. HARRIS to				
Tyler . . .	13	—	0	0
W. Meacock . .	18	—	5	400
M. Meacock . .	29	—	5	20
R. Meacock . .	1	—	3	6
Porch . . .	3	6	0	2
E. Porch . . .	2	—	0	0
J. Porch . . .	—	4	3	350
Fermoy . . .	—	11	0	60
Gurney . . .	—	11	0	0
Downs . . .	1	6	3	200
From WADE to				
Mays . . .	1	1	2	500
From J. MUNDY to				
Matthews . . .	—	4	2	0
From BREWSTER to				
M. Brewfter . .	—	11	0	0
From LEE's Puftules to				
Baker . . .	29	—	3	140
Caterer . . .	15	—	5	8
R. Featherftone . .	12	—	3	40
C. Featherftone . .	9	—	3	120
Porter . . .	5	—	0	9

	Age, Years.	Months	Days of Illnes.	No. of Puftules.
From LEE's Puftules to				
J. Porter . . .	1	6	1	12
J. Jennings . .	5	—	1	30
C. Jennings . .	3	—	1	30
W. Jennings . .	1	1	0	9
Mansfield . . .	1	6	2	12
S. Wybrow . .	6	—	2	300
S. Baker . . .	1	1	3	25
J. Gofs . . .	2	8	1	0
W. Gofs . . .	—	8	2	30
Odell . . .	—	9	3	90
Murphield . . .	—	6	2	0
From DALKINS to				
Sharp . . .	—	4	2	0
From WAITE to				
T. Jennings . .	1	6	0	0
Kitchen . . .	5	—	1	0
S. Pluckrofe . .	4	—	2	0
T. Pluckrofe . .	—	10	2	0
Rout . . .	—	6	1	20
W. Houghton . .	2	6	1	0
From SWANNELL to				
Mickland . . .	—	2	0	3
Fergufon . . .	—	7	1	7
Goddard . . .	1	—	2	0
Roberts . . .	—	9	1	0
Gran . . .	—	6	1	0
Benfon . . .	—	8	2	0
Floaks . . .	—	2	1	2

	Age, Years.	Months	Days of Illness.	No. of Pustules.
From M. GILBERT to				
Welch . . .	15	—	3	100
Rowley . . .	—	3	2	25
A. Waite . . .	17	—	4	10
Tarbotts . . .	1	1	2	600
S. Tarbotts . .	3	3	4	300
Bell . . .	—	3	3	250
From S. HOPES to				
Snell . . .	17	—	2	200
I. Houghton . .	32	—	3	200
Stedman . . .	—	5	3	60
M. Broadwood . .	—	6	2	150
W. Broadwood . .	—	6	2	200
Sorrell . . .	4	11	4	500
S. Sorrell . .	6	—	1	1
Underwood . .	—	9	2	105
From ELLIKIN to				
G. Cooke . .	2	2	3	20
Coſtin . . .	—	5	2	0
From REYNOLDS to				
Walford . . .	—	6	2	600
From WADE to				
Wentworth . .	1	8	3	500
Gibſon . . .	—	8	0	0
Liſter . . .	—	5	0	0
Wooden . . .	1	4	4	0
Smart . . .	6	—	2	0
Taylor . . .	1	—	1	200

	Age, Years.	Months	Days of Illness.	No. of Pustules.
From WADE to				
Arnold	—	5	3	0
Turvey	—	3	2	12
Guilder	2	3	2	0
Gallop	—	2	2	0
Stanny	2	2	4	2
Moore	—	4	0	0
M. Moore	2	6	1	0
From OLIPHANT to				
Abfalom	—	7	1	0
From M. FORD to				
Clark	2	4	3	0
Cox	1	7	2	0
Sandaw	—	2	0	0
From J. ROBERTS to				
T. Roberts	3	—	3	0
From KITCHEN to				
T. Fofter	5	—	2	5
J. Fofter	1		1	2
M. Fofter	1		1	24
S. Gobby	27	—	2	20
W. Gobby	5	—	0	2
J. Gobby	—	6	3	0
Putney	—	7	2	0
Bufh	1	7	1	0
E. Franklin	3		2	0
S. Franklin	—	8	0	0
Neat	2		2	9
Hicks	3		2	0

	Age, Years.	Months	Days of Illness.	No. of Pustules.
From KITCHEN to				
More	—	5	0	0
Barker	6	—	2	6
North	2	—	3	0
Cowland	1	3	3	12
Harrison	—	8	1	5
R. Lawyer	36	—	1	1
E. Lawyer	3	6	1	7
F. Lawyer	4	6	0	0
M. Lawyer	1	—	0	0
E. Dunn	5		0	0
F. Dunn	2	6	0	0
T. Dunn	—	3	2	6
N. Collop	9	—	1	0
J. Collop	7	—	1	0
A. Collop	3	—	1	0
E. Collop	—	5	0	0
T. Wiggins	7		0	0
W. Wiggins	4		0	0
P. Wiggins	1	6	0	0
Ruffles	19	—	2	6
Bridges	—	1	0	0
From I. BARRETT to				
I. Mitchell	6	—	2	100
P. Mitchell	4	—	2	50
T. Mitchell	2	—	2	26
From COOK to				
E. Chapman	12	—	2	27
M. Chapman	9	—	3	67

	Age, Years.	Months	Days of Illnefs.	No. of Puftules.
From Cook to				
Good . . .	13	—.	4	400
From Styles to				
Edwards . . .	18	—	3	0
From Talbot to				
Brandrom . . .	12	—	0	0
From Caterer to				
Stapler . . .	22	—	4	300
Marfham . . .	17	—	4	43
Waller . . .	18	—	3	15
Wall . . .	8	—	3	200
R. Johnfton . .	—	3	2	0
Fletcher . . .	—	6	3	500
From Bradley's Puftules to				
Vaughan . . .	—	5	2	12
Vethall . . .	-	4	3	200
Hope . . .	—	6	4	100
Mafterfon . .	—	5	2	20
Green . . .	2	4	3	30
Lutman . . .	1	—	2	20
Roberts . . .	—	4	3	450
Starbuck . . .	—	5	2	20
M. Phillips . .	2	2	3	500
S. Phillips . .	3	11	3	5
Wicks . . .	—	4	2	36
Terry . . .	—	3	2	8
Sheriff . . .	7	—	3	34
Steers . . .	13	—	3	40

	Age, Years.	Months	Days of Illness.	No. of Pustules.
From I. Houghton to				
S. Houghton . .	19	—	0	0
W. Houghton . .	58	—	0	0
Jolly . . .	1	8	0	0
From T. Pluckrose to				
Lineau . . .	12	—	3	3
Wooland . . .	2		0	0
From Kitchen to				
Kettridge . .	16	—	1	3
Raymond . . .	1	—	1	3
From I. Harwood to				
A. Harris . .	26	—	4	100
M. Harris . .	—	1	4	500
S. Harris . .	4	6	5	50
W. Harris . .	5	6	2	25
G. Harris . .	2	6	1	5
S. Boyton . .	8		4	700
E. Boyton . .	6		3	600
J. Boyton . .	3		3	350
From Talbot to				
Lemare . . .	—	6	3	60
Williams . . .	—	9	4	650
English . . .	1	3	2	100
Churchman . .	—	3	4	30
Hunt . . .	1	2	4	700
Whitburn . .		9	4	430
Chartau . . .		10	4	17
Callen . . .		8	3	75
Ruffel . . .	—	5	4	15

	Age, Years.	Months	Days of Illnefs.	No. of Puftules.
From TALBOT to				
E. Ruffel	3	6	3	12
Knight	—	8	3	500
Richardfon	—	6	2	200
Johnfton	1	7	3	150
From J. GOSS to				
Blinkinhorn	—	2	0	0
Millward	—	7	0	5
Haywood	1	8	4	46
A. Godden	1	—	2	300
W. Godden	3	—	3	650
Jones	—	6	0	0
Paradife	3	—	3	50
Kelly	2	—	0	100
Hales	—	6	4	500
I. Mountain	4	6	2	300
M. Mountain	2	—	2	150
A. Mountain	1	—	1	75
From BREWSTER to				
Barnett	1	1		
Balling	—	9	2	6
Upton	1	9	3	0
Fenn	1	1	2	0
Hilliard	—	6	0	0
White	1	4	1	0
From W. MEACOCK to				
Weftbrook	—	3	0	0
From E. CHAPMAN to				
Hider	—	2	1	0

	Age Years.	Months	Days of Illness.	No. of Pustules.
From E. Chapman to				
Hughes	1	8	3	12
C. Hughes	—	5	2	4
From M. Chapman to				
Sharp	18	0	3	30
Calburn	16	—	3	12
Ledger	—	4	2	50
Vautin	1	—	1	2
M'Kennish	4	3	2	150
Wright	—	7	3	10
Rance	—	2	0	0
From Ruffles to				
Thornton	17	—	1	0
Boreham	16	—	2	3
Hill	—	5	1	0
Towler	1	3	1	0
French	—	11	0	0
Breſtley	—	8	0	0
Thomas	—	4	1	0
Richardſon	—	9	0	0
Morgan	—	5	0	0
From A. Waite to				
Wood	22	—	4	6
Young	16	—	2	0
Norman	12	—	2	0
M. Bartlett	—	11	1	20
Aſkew	—	3	0	15
Clark	—	9	0	0

Thofe who are acquainted with the hiftory of the Cow-pox, will no doubt be furprifed to find from the preceding cafes, that puftules have frequently been the confequence of the Inoculation of this difeafe. Indeed, when I firft obferved a puftular eruption upon Buckland, (Cafe 3d) the occurrence being wholly unexpected, I was not without apprehenfion that the lancet which was employed in his inoculation might have had fome particles of variolous matter adhering to it. But this fufpicion was foon removed; for, upon enquiry, I found that all the lancets which I had ufed on the 21ft of January, were then made ufe of for the firft time fince they had been ground by the cutler.

Among the patients inoculated for the Cow-pox during the firft week in which I obtained the matter of this difeafe, feveral were fo circumftanced as to be afterwards

s   conftantly

conſtantly expoſed to the infection of the
Small-pox. Having then had no proof that the
progreſs of the infection of the former would
ſuperſede that of the latter, I uſed the pre-
caution to inoculate the patients with variolous matter on the fifth day after that taken
from the cow had been inſerted. This led
ſome medical gentlemen to ſuppoſe that the
matter locally formed in the arm from the
firſt inoculation, might be variolated by the
progreſs of the ſecond inoculation in the other
arm, and that conſequently the matter generated in the Cow-pox tumour with which
others were inoculated, would produce a hybrid diſeaſe, and not the genuine Cow-pox.
But as the matter employed in the Cow-pox
inoculations was always taken before the con-
ſtitution could be affected by the variolous
matter, and during the time that both inoculations were merely local diſeaſes, I appre-
hend

hend its effects would be the same as if the variolous inoculation had not taken place. Nay, had this not been the case, but had several patients been inoculated with matter taken from the Cow-pox tumour on the arm of Jane Collingridge, after both the inoculations were supposed to have affected the constitution for several days, neither facts nor analogy lead us to believe that the matter thus obtained would produce any other disease than that of its own species, or that its specific morbid quality would be changed by entering into combination with the virus of the Small-pox. The general character of the tumour formed by the inoculation of the Small-pox, is very different from that of the Cow-pox; and though on the same day a person be inoculated in one arm with the matter of the Cow-pox, and in the other with that of the Small-pox, yet both tumours preserve their

respective

respective characteristic appearances throughout the whole course of the disease. This is certainly a strong proof that the two diseases, in respect to their local action, continue separate and distinct.

Twenty-eight patients were on the same day inoculated with the matter of Cow-pox, and that of the Small-pox, mixed together in equal quantities, in order to try which would prevail, or if it were possible to produce a hybrid disease by a union of both. The result was, that in more than one half of the patients thus inoculated, the local affection distinctly assumed the characters of the Cow-pox; in the others it more resembled the Small-pox, but in none of them was there much indisposition, or many pustules.

At the request of Dr. Jenner, I transmitted to him, in Gloucestershire, some of the Cow-pox matter, from the patients then under

my

my care, which he ufed for the purpofe of inoculation: after a trial of it, he informed me, that " the rife, progrefs, and termination of the puftule, created by this virus on the arm, was exactly that of the true uncontaminated Cow-pox." The matter fent was taken from the arm of Ann Bumpus, who had 310 puftules, all of which fuppurated; yet with the matter of this ftock, Dr. Jenner inoculated twenty, and another gentleman, in the fame county, 140 perfons, without producing any puftules which maturated.

This fact would appear to confirm an opinion entertained by Dr. Jenner. In his fecond publication on the variolæ vaccinæ he feems difpofed to attribute the puftules which fo often attended this difeafe in London and it's vicinity, to fome peculiar influence of the town air. But of the cafes which I have ftated, feveral were thofe of patients who were

inoculated

inoculated eight miles diftance from London:
yet thefe patients, in the proportion of about
one in five, had an eruption. And at a fmall
village, ftill farther from London, eighteen
perfons were inoculated with fimilar matter,
in all of whom it produced puftules.

The 27th Cafe alfo affords decifive evidence, that the matter employed in it was
that of the Cow-pox, for Jewel had undergone the Small-pox when a child; yet the
inoculation excited febrile fymptoms of two
or three days duration, and the tumour which
was produced upon her arm, did not begin to
fcab till the 13th day.

Having now, I prefume, given fufficient rea-
fons for eftablifhing the point for which they
have been adduced, I fhall proceed to enquire
how far the effects of the Cow-pox, upon
the human fubject, feem to differ from or
correfpond with, thofe of the Small-pox,
when communicated by inoculation.

The

The vaccine difeafe, as it has lately been called, affords a ftriking example, and perhaps the only one yet difcovered, of a diforder which can be transferred from brute animals to man, and carried back again from him to the brute. A remarkable inftance of this is related at page 62, which fhows, that the matter of the Cow-pox, as reproduced by inoculation in the human animal, and inferted into the teat of a Cow, produced the difeafe. Similar attempts were alfo made with variolous matter, which had no effect; hence in this refpect thefe two morbid poifons appear to differ. The Cow-pox alfo differs from the Small-pox in acting upon the conftitutions of thofe who have undergone the latter difeafe, as was fully exemplified in the cafe of Frances Jewel. However, I am difpofed to think, that the matter of the Cow-pox is not fo capable of affecting perfons, who have had the Small-

pox

pox, as has been reprefented. I made feveral trials to inoculate this difeafe in patients at the Hofpital, who were recovering from a full eruption of the natural Small-pox, but in no inftance did any tumour appear on the arm; neither does the infertion of the vario- lous matter, in fuch cafes, excite the leaft inflammation in the fkin. It is probable, therefore, that the matter of the Cow-pox, like that of the Small-pox, does not manifeft any local action upon perfons who have lately un- dergone the variolous difeafe. If a perfon has cafually received the infection of the Small-pox, and be inoculated with variolous matter three or four days before the eruptive fymptoms fupervene, the inoculated part does not tumify, as in other cafes, but becomes a fimple puftule: on the contrary, if a perfon has been inoculated, and the progrefs of the inoculation be fo far advanced that the patient is

within

within one day of the approach of the eruptive
fever, and be then inoculated a fecond time,
the tumour produced, from the fecond inoculation, will become nearly as extenfive as the
firft, and be in a ftate of fuppuration a few
hours after the fever commences. Hence it
appears, that the procefs of variolation in the
natural and in the inoculated Small-pox, is
different. The Cow-pox, in every cafe with
which we are acquainted, has been intro-
duced into the human conftitution through
the medium of external local inflammation,
and is therefore to be confidered as an inoculated difeafe: the virus of it feems alfo to
affect a fimilar mode of action, and to be
governed by the fame laws as that of the
Small-pox. Thus if a perfon be alternately
inoculated with variolous matter, and with
that of the Cow-pox every day till fever is
excited, all the inoculations make a progrefs;

T   and

and as foon as the whole fyftem becomes difordered, they appear to be all equally advanced in maturation. However, the local
tumour excited from the inoculation of the
Cow-pox, is commonly of a different appearance from that which is the confequence of
inoculation with variolous matter; for if the
inoculation be performed by-a fimple puncture, the confequent tumour, in the proportion
of three times out of four, or more, affumes a
form completely circular, and it continues
circumfcribed, with its edges elevated, and
well defined, and its furface flat throughout
every ftage of the difeafe; while that which
is produced from variolous matter, either pre-
ferves a puftular form, or fpreads along the
fkin, and becomes angulated and irregular,
or disfigured by numerous veficulæ.

Another diftinction, ftill more general and
decifive, is to be drawn from the contents of
the

the Cow-pox tumour; for the fluid it forms, unlefs from fome accidental circumftance, very rarely becomes puriform, and the fcab which fucceeds is of a harder texture, exhibits a fmoother furface, and differs in its colour from that which is formed by the concretion of pus. All the appearances here defcribed, however, do not conftantly attend the difeafe, but are fometimes fo much changed, they can in no refpect be diftinguifhed from thofe which arife from the inoculation of the Small-pox. When the difeafe thus deviates from its ufual appearance at the inoculated part, its effects upon the conftitution, have commonly, though not always, been felt more feverely than where the tumour was diftinctly cha-racterifed.

As I have now pointed out the principal circumftances in which the two difeafes ufu-ally differ in their local effects, I fhall proceed

to

to examine them in a more important point
of view, and to compare their general effects
upon the conftitution, in order, if poffible, to
afcertain, from the facts already adduced, whether or not the inoculation of the vaccine difeafe produces a milder diftemper, and of lefs
dangerous confequences to the patient, than
that of the Small-pox. For if it be an efta-
blifhed fact, as I prefume it is, that thofe
who have undergone the former difeafe are
thereby rendered fecure againft the effects
of the latter, it only remains to be proved, in
order to make the former be generally adopted,
that the diforder which attends the Cow-pox
is alfo lefs fevere and lefs fatal than the other.
The number of cafes of Cow-pox, inoculated
under my direction, have amounted to about
600, but all thefe could not be included in
the table, as at the time it was printed, the
difeafe, in many patients, was not far enough
advanced

advanced to give the refult; and to thefe may be added others who did not give proper attendance, and alfo fome whofe names I am not permitted to make public.

The table, however, contains a fufficient number of cafes to enable the medical reader to form a tolerably correct judgment refpecting the difeafe; and from-confidering what would have probably been the effects of an equal number of cafes of variolous inoculation, he may draw his own conclufions. But before this is done, I have to obferve, that fince the table was compofed, an infant at the breaft died on the eleventh day after the Cow-pox matter had been inferted in its arm. In this folitary fatal cafe, the local tumour was very inconfiderable, and the eruptive fymptoms took place on the feventh day, when the child was attacked with fits of the fpafmodic kind, which recurred at fhort intervals with
increafed

increafed violence, and carried it off at the time above mentioned, after an eruption of eighty or one hundred puftules.

It appears, therefore, that out of about 500 cafes of the inoculated Cow-pox, one proved fatal, and the preceding table fhows that in fome others the difeafe, from the number of the puftules, was of formidable feverity; while, on the other hand, a very large proportion of the patients were fcarcely difordered from the inoculation, and had no puftules.

Were I enabled to ftate a number of cafes of variolous inoculation, equal to thofe given above, and reduced to a fimilar tabular form, the comparative magnitude of the two difeafes might be eftimated with tolerable precifion. It is evident, however, that the matter of the vaccine difeafe has generally produced much fewer puftules, and lefs indifpo-

tion

tion than that of the Small-pox; for it appears from the preceding ftatement, that about two-fifths of all the perfons inoculated for the variolæ vaccinæ, had no puftules, and that in not more than a fourth part of them was there experienced any perceptible diforder of the conftitution. But it muft be acknowledged, that in feveral inftances, the Cow-pox has proved a very fevere difeafe. In three or four cafes, out of 500, the patient has been in confiderable danger, and one child, as I have already obferved, actually died under the effects of the difeafe. Now, if it be admitted, that at an average, one of 500 will die of the inoculated Cow-pox, I confefs I fhould not be difpofed to introduce this difeafe into the Inoculation Hofpital, becaufe, out of the laft 5000 cafes of variolous inoculation, the number of deaths has not exceeded the proportion of one in 600. But I am

inclined

inclined to think, that if the matter of the Cow-pox, ufed for the purpofe of inoculation, were only taken from thofe in whom the difeafe appeared in a very mild form, the refult would be more favourable than in the ftatement here given. For though it has occafionally happened, that the matter taken from the arm of a patient, in whom the diforder neither produced fever nor eruption, has in others produced both ; yet ftill it has much more commonly had the effect of exciting a milder difeafe than the matter of the puftules, or than that which was obtained from a patient who had the difeafe in a fevere manner, as may be feen by an examination of the table.

Thus we find, that out of fixty-two perfons, who were inoculated with the puftule matter, fifty-feven had an eruption; and thofe who received the difeafe from any of thefe fifty-feven patients, appear alfo to have had

puftules

puſtules in nearly the ſame proportion. I may alſo remark, that the diſeaſe, before noticed as proving fatal to a patient, was excited from matter of this deſcription, and taken from Talbot, (ſee p. 134.) Whence it appears, that the Cow-pox, from certain circumſtances, is not only liable to loſe the characters which diſtinguiſh it from the Small-pox, but alſo to continue to propagate itſelf under this new and caſual modification. The vaccine variolæ, and the human variolæ, ought therefore to be conſidered as only varieties of the ſame diſeaſe, rather than as diſtinct ſpecies.

One important advantage which the Cow-pox is ſuppoſed to have over the Small-pox is that the former is not a contagious diſeaſe, and not to be propagated by the effluvia of perſons infected with it. This is certainly true when the diſorder is confined to the inoculated part,

U   but

but where is produces numerous puftules upon the body, the exhalation they fend forth are capable of infecting others in the fame manner as the Small-pox. Two inftances of cafual infection in this way have lately fallen under my obfervation; in one the difeafe was fevere, and the eruption confluent; in the other the difeafe was mild, and the puftules few.

It has been afferted, that perfons have had the Small-pox after having been affected with the Cow-pox ; and fome facts have been publifhed with a view to fhow that inftances of this kind have actually happened. But all thefe, as far as I have feen, have been very defective in not affording fufficient proof, that the affcction fuppofed to have been the Cow-pox, was in reality that difeafe. On the other hand, the inftances which have been brought forward to prove that thofe who had under-gone the genuine Cow-pox refifted the infec-tion

tion of the Small-pox, are unqueftionably
decifive, and fufficiently numerous to eftablifh
the fact in the moft fatisfactory manner. This
circumftance then appears to be as much a
general law of the fyftem, as that a perfon
having had the Small-pox is thereby rendered
unfufceptible of receiving the difeafe a fecond
time. For of all the patients whom I inoculated with variolous matter, after they had
paffed through the Cow-pox, amounting to
upwards of 400, none were affected with
the Small-pox; and it may be remarked, that
nearly a fourth part of this number was fo
flightly affected with the Cow-pox, that it
neither produced any perceptible indifpofition,
nor puftules.

We have been told, that the Cow-pox
tumour has frequently produced eryfipelatous
inflammation, and phagedenic ulceration; but
the inoculated part has not ulcerated in any

of

of the cases which have been under my care, nor have I obferved inflammation to occafion any inconvenience, except in one inftance, where it was foon fubdued by the application of aqua lithargyri acetati. It fhould feem then, that the advantages to be derived from fubftituting the Cow-pox for the Small-pox, muft be directly in proportion to the greater mildnefs of the former, than the latter difeafe.

PUBLISHED by the fame AUTHOR,

The HISTORY of the INOCULATION of the SMALL-POX in GREAT BRITAIN;
Comprehending a Review of all the Publications on the Subject; with an Experimental Inquiry into the relative Advantages of every Meafure which has been deemed neceffary in the Procefs of Inoculation.—8vo. 7s. boards.
The Second Volume, which concludes the Work, is nearly ready for the Prefs.

MEDICAL BOTANY,

Containing fyftematic and general Defcriptions, with Plates, of all the Medicinal Plants, indigenous and exotic, comprehended in the Catalogues of the MATERIA MEDICA, as publifhed by the Royal Colleges of Phyficians of LONDON and EDINBURGH. Accompanied with a circumftantial Detail of their Medicinal Effects, and of the Difeafes in which they have been moft fuc-cefsfully employed. In 3 vols. 4to.——To which is added, a Supplement, or Part the Second; containing Plates, with De-fcriptions of moft of the principal Medicinal Plants not included in the Collegiate Pharmacopœias of London and Edinburgh.— 2l. 19s. in boards.—Coloured, 7l. 1s. 6d.

Printed in the United States
By Bookmasters